Esophageal Disease and Testing

Esophageal Disease and Testing

Cedric G. Bremner
University of Southern California
Los Angeles, California, U.S.A.

Tom R. DeMeester
University of Southern California
Los Angeles, California, U.S.A.

James E. Huprich
Mayo Clinic
Rochester, Minnesota, U.S.A.

Ross M. Bremner
University of Southern California
Los Angeles, California, U.S.A.

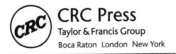

CRC Press
Taylor & Francis Group
Boca Raton London New York

CRC Press is an imprint of the
Taylor & Francis Group, an **informa** business

CRC Press
Taylor & Francis Group
6000 Broken Sound Parkway NW, Suite 300
Boca Raton, FL 33487-2742

First issued in paperback 2019

© 2005 by Taylor & Francis Group, LLC
CRC Press is an imprint of Taylor & Francis Group, an Informa business

No claim to original U.S. Government works

ISBN-13: 978-0-8247-2842-7 (hbk)
ISBN-13: 978-0-367-39224-6 (pbk)

Visit the Taylor & Francis Web site at
http://www.taylorandfrancis.com

and the CRC Press Web site at
http://www.crcpress.com

Library of Congress Cataloging-in-Publication Data

Catalog record is available from the Library of Congress

Preface

Techniques to investigate the esophagus have improved and expanded to meet the need of an explosion in the prevalence and interest in esophageal diseases, notably gastroesophageal reflux disease and adenocarcinoma at the cardia. Newer techniques have evolved to improve the understanding of the pathophysiology of esophageal diseases, and in many respects reinforce existing concepts rather than making them obsolete.

An adequate investigation of esophageal anatomy and function requires radiological, endoscopic, and manometric techniques. The results of these tests although not always conclusive, provide sufficient comprehension of the patients' complaints to at least choose the right direction for effective surgical management. Often insights are obtained that could not have been thought of had the tests not been done. The more detailed our understanding, the more effective our therapy. Radiology of the esophagus provides visualization of any structural changes, such as strictures, cancer, diverticula, and hernias. Moreover, the extent of the abnormality is more clearly defined before the passage of an endoscope. Endoscopy is essential to detect superficial lesions, Barrett's esophagus, early cancer, and to provide a grading of the structural geometry of the cardia. Ineffective esophageal body motility, and/or a hypo- or hypertensive lower esophageal sphincter can only be diagnosed by manometric studies. Failure to do manometry on unexplained dysphagia may preclude a patient from the benefits of appropriate treatment.

Esophageal impedance studies are useful in defining bolus transport, and to clarify the nature of regurgitation. Combined with a pH probe, impedance studies can distinguish between acid and alkaline reflux episodes. The Bilitec probe may be worthwhile in some situations to distinguish between bile and nonbilious alkaline fluid such as saliva, whereas the recent introduction of a tubeless pH probe makes the 24 h pH monitoring comfortable for the patient.

This book has been compiled by a group of clinicians who have made dedicated studies on the esophagus for many years, and has been compiled to give a clear description about the use and interpretation of each test.

We hope that you will enjoy reading this book as much as we have enjoyed compiling it.

Cedric G. Bremner
Tom R. DeMeester
James E. Huprich
Ross M. Bremner

v

Contents

1

Radiology of the Esophagus

1. INTRODUCTION

Soon after the discovery of X-rays, near the end of the 20th century, the new science found a use in medicine. Contrast studies of the gastrointestinal (GI) tract were one of the first clinical applications. Until the middle of the last century contrast studies were virtually the only way to evaluate GI tract. During the last century, much of our understanding of GI function and disease was derived from these early studies. In the past 30–40 years endoscopy has largely replaced barium studies for the evaluation of mucosal disease of the GI tract. Although barium studies are not as sensitive as endoscopy for diagnosis of mucosal disease, by virtue of their simplicity, relative safety, and low cost, the barium exam can provide complimentary as well as unique information about esophageal disease. In the evaluation of esophageal function, the barium swallow competes very effectively with manometry (1,2). Furthermore, when compared with esophageal manometry, barium swallow technique is easier to interpret and does not require additional expensive equipment or specialized training.

The following sections on imaging will primarily cover the use of the barium swallow in evaluating patients with esophageal disease. Our purpose is not to provide a comprehensive discussion of all aspects of esophageal disease but to emphasize the most important points through images. Minimal attention will be given to evaluating pharyngeal disease and the reader should refer to the bibliography for additional information on this subject (3,4).

Newer imaging techniques such as computed tomography (CT), magnetic resonance (MR) imaging, and positron emission tomography (PET) have special roles in esophageal disease and are likely to become more important in the future (5–9). When appropriate, their use will be discussed.

The following is a list of general indications for a barium swallow. The sensitivity and specificity of the barium exam varies greatly depending on the suspected condition.

- Globus sensation
- Dysphagia
- Regurgitation
- Gastroesophageal reflux disease (GERD)
- Noncardiac chest pain
- Esophageal neoplasm
- Suspected postoperative complications

2. TECHNIQUE

The technique of barium examination described in this section is designed to detect both anatomical and functional abnormalities of the esophagus. We have found this technique useful in evaluating thousands of patients as a part of their initial workup. When performing the exam we do not deviate significantly from the protocol from patient to patient because we believe that our ability to detect abnormalities depends on eliminating variables introduced by variations in exam technique. As one will discover, the exam is comprehensive but requires significant practice to achieve consistent results.

2.1. General Comments

2.1.1. Motion Recording

The act of swallowing is a dynamic process and, as such, its evaluation cannot be adequately assessed with static films alone. All studies should include videotape recording of the exam (S-VHS format) as indicated in the exam protocol. A separate cassette for each patient can be used so that subsequent exams can be added. The tapes are not only provide a permanent record of the exams but also used for patient education when discussing treatment options.

2.1.2. Large Image Intensifier

The esophagus is 24–27 cm long (10.5 in.), excluding the pharynx. Optimally, one would like to visualize the entire esophagus and lower pharynx during swallowing so as to not miss significant events while focusing on a specific area (e.g., stasis behind an ineffective peristaltic contraction, airway penetration, transient filling of a diverticulum, etc.). The largest field of view available on older fluoroscopic units is 9 in., which will only allow visualization of a portion of the esophagus at one time. Because of these limitations a large image intensifier ($\geq$ 14 in.) is better suited for examination. With a large image intensifier centered over the aortic arch one can visualize the entire esophagus from the UES (C5–6 level) to the gastroesophageal junction (GEJ).

2.1.3. Examination of the Stomach and Duodenum

It is becoming increasingly appreciated that the stomach plays a major role in the pathogenesis of GERD. A significant portion of patients with GERD have gastric abnormalities, which may alter treatment. It is therefore important, especially in GERD patients, to examine the stomach and duodenum as well as the esophagus to look for evidence of previous surgery, peptic disease, signs of delayed gastric emptying, etc.

It has also been shown that dysphagia may be associated with gastric cancer. Therefore, if the examination of the esophagus fails to detect an abnormality to explain the patient's dysphagia the stomach should also be examined (10).

2.2. Exam Details

1. *Videotape lateral mouth/neck to include mouth, soft palate, and pharynx. Have patient swallow single boluses of high density barium. Stay in one place—do not pan.*

The symptoms of dysphagia are often poorly localized (11); therefore, it is important to always examine the pharynx and the esophagus. In addition, there is an increased incidence of associated pharyngeal abnormalities in patients with esophageal disorders, particularly GERD (12,13).

It is always tempting to follow the swallowed bolus but this is distracting when reviewing the tape, so stay in one place and do not pan. Use high density barium to optimally coat the surfaces. If airway penetration or aspiration is suspected or observed, barium of various consistencies should be used. No need to take spot films.

2. *Videotape lateral neck to include C5–6 while patient takes several swallows of high density barium from cup. (It helps if the shoulders are kept oblique, with head in lateral position to penetrate cervicothoracic junction adequately.) Stay in one place—do not pan.*

Use this view to search for Zenker's diverticula, webs and cricopharyngeal abnormalities, etc. The cricopharyngeus is usually located near the C5–6 level. If this area is obscured in the lateral view by the shoulders, placing the patient in a shallow oblique position may help to visualize the lower cervical region. Again, do not pan—stay in one place.

3. *Take upright air-contrast spot films of entire esophagus.*

We have found that the best way to get consistent distension is to give effervescent crystals in a small amount of water followed by two large gulps of high density barium. Immediately take the spots films, as a healthy esophageal body will collapse quickly. At best, good distension will be obtained in 80% of the films in normal patients. Use a 14 in. film to include the entire esophagus. This large format also provides much better mucosal detail when compared with digital spots.

4. *Take upright spot films of mucosal relief of distal collapsed esophagus.*

This can be performed when the esophagus is collapsed after the air-contrast films. Again, use a three-on-one format with a 14 in. cassette centered to include the entire esophagus, but do not exclude the GEJ. We have found this to be the best technique to detect reflux esophagitis.

5. *Take upright videotape passage of bolus through GEJ without panning.*

This view is used along with the equivalent supine view (see 9) to estimate whether a hiatal hernia is reducible or not (see Section 4). Mucosal rings, stricture, or other segmental narrowing lesions may not be visible in the upright position (14). Always use the recumbent images to diagnose these abnormalities.

6. *In prone right anterior oblique position ask patient to swallow 10 cc boluses of low density barium. Instruct patient to swallow the entire volume at once and not to divide it up. Videotape tail of bolus looking for stasis. Repeat for a total of five swallows (if the first three demonstrate normal transport, stop).*

The patient is placed in the prone slightly right anterior oblique position with the right arm at the side. Have the assistant fill a 10 cc disposable syringe with low density barium. This can be attached to the female end of IV extension tubing that has been cut to a length of a few inches. Instruct the patient to swallow the entire bolus at once and not to swallow again until the next bolus is given. This assures that the bolus will distend the walls of the esophagus and sustain the peristalsis as well as prevent deglutitive inhibition from suppressing peristalsis giving the erroneous impression of failed peristalsis. It is important to follow the tail of the bolus (i.e., head of the peristaltic wave) from the cervicothoracic junction to the stomach. A large image intensifier will allow one to see the entire bolus and help detect subsequent swallows. Look for significant stasis of contrast in the esophagus as a result of ineffective or failed peristaltic contractions. Significant stasis is defined as a column of barium that is dense enough so that the underlying structures cannot be seen through it. If the first three swallows result in complete clearance, motility is probably normal and can be stopped after three swallows. If significant stasis occurs record a total of five swallows.

7. *In prone right anterior oblique position ask patient to swallow a cup of barium as rapidly as possible. Obtain 14 in. × 14 in. three-on-one films to include entire esophagus when maximally filled.*

Be sure to wait until the entire esophagus is filled with barium from top to bottom. Encourage the patient to drink rapidly (patients are instructed to drink as fast as they can). These images are the best methods of demonstrating areas of narrowing and extrinsic compression. They are also useful for measuring maximal esophageal diameter (MED, discussed later).

8. *In prone right anterior oblique videotape a single bolus of barium passing through GEJ.*

9. *In supine, slightly left posterior oblique position, videotape a bolus of barium passing through the GEJ.*

This is the best method for evaluating a hiatal hernia. Compare the appearance and size of hernia with that seen on upright view to determine if the hernia is reducible. This is also a good view to evaluate the emptying of hernia into stomach (hiatal flow).

3. NORMAL APPEARANCE AND VARIANTS

The fully distended esophagus has a smooth, featureless appearance on air-contrast images (Fig. 1.1). When the esophagus collapses the redundant mucosa produces smooth longitudinal folds up to 3–4 mm in diameter (Fig. 1.2). The folds can be followed for several centimeters and should not be discontinuous. The contour of the esophageal wall on full-column films should be smooth without any irregularity (Fig. 1.3). Occasionally tertiary contractions may produce contour irregularities. The transient nature of

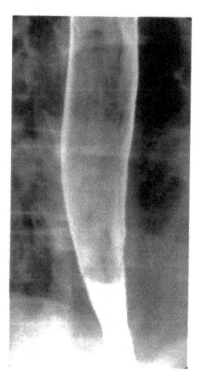

Figure 1.1 Normal air-contrast image of esophagus. Mucosa appears smooth and featureless.

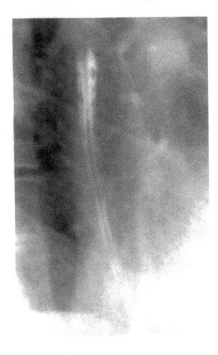

Figure 1.2 Normal mucosal relief. Collapsed esophagus with barium caught in smooth longitudinal
folds measuring <3–4 mm.

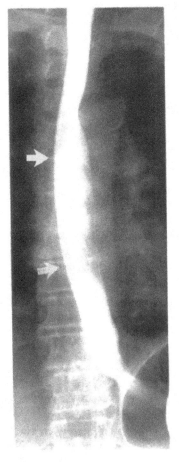

Figure 1.3 Normal full column view. Margins of maximally
filled esophagus are smooth (arrows).

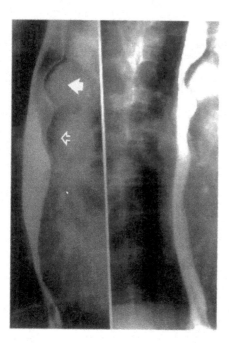

Figure 1.4 Normal impressions on esophageal body. Oblique view of mid-esophagus shows extrinsic impressions produced by aorta (closed arrow) and left mainstem bronchus (open arrow).

these irregularities should be obvious fluoroscopically. Fixed irregularities, no matter how subtle, are almost always abnormal.

Normal structures produce extrinsic impressions on the esophagus and need to be differentiated from pathological conditions. The transverse aorta and left mainstem bronchus indent the middle third of the distended esophagus and produce eccentric impressions on the filled esophagus (Fig. 1.4). These normal extrinsic impressions become exaggerated if the esophagus is dilated as in a motility disorder. The esophageal hiatus produces a circumferential narrowing of the esophagus as it passes into the abdomen. This narrowing increases during inspiration—a fact that is helpful in locating the transition from the intrathoracic to the abdominal segment of the esophagus. With the patient in the prone oblique position and with the head turned, the trachea may also produce an oblique extrinsic impression at the level of the thoracic inlet. Occasionally an enlarged left atrium will produce posterior deviation of the esophagus in the lateral view. A peristaltic contraction can give the impression of an extrinsic defect if one only looks at the static images. Extrinsic impressions other than those described above should be viewed with suspicion and may indicate pathology.

The esophagus is uniform in caliber throughout its length except in the distal portion. Just above the hiatus the esophagus widens slightly. This area is called the esophageal ampulla and may be confused with a small hiatal hernia (15).

3.1. Normal Variants

Glycogenic acanthosis produces multiple subtle nodular mucosal elevations due to the accumulation of cytoplasmic glycogen in squamous epithelial cells (Fig. 1.5). This condition is fairly common, especially in the elderly, and must be differentiated from pathology such as monilial esophagitis (Fig. 1.6).

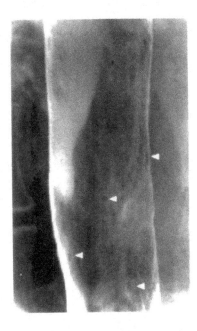

Figure 1.5 Glycogenic achanthosis. Multiple tiny poly-
poid elevations of the esophageal mucosa (arrowheads).
(With permission from Mayo Foundation, Johnson CD.
Alimentary Tract Imaging: A Teaching File. Mosby-
Yearbook, 1993.)

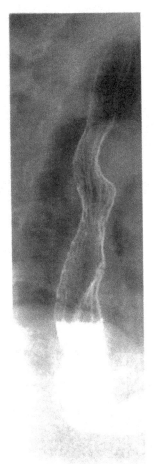

Figure 1.6 Scleroderma with monilial esophagitis producing
plaque-like elevations on the mucosal folds. Infection likely due
to marked stasis from severe esophageal hypomotility; hiatal
hernia with stricture at GEJ visible distally.

Occasionally, fine evenly spaced transverse folds can be seen in the esophageal body and are referred to as "feline esophagus" (Fig. 1.7). This deformity is probably the result of contraction of the longitudinal muscle that causes infolding of the mucosa producing a finely corrugated appearance. This condition has been described in reflux disease (16) but is more commonly seen in normal patients.

During the performance of double-contrast exam, undissolved gas crystals or air bubbles may adhere to the esophageal wall to produce tiny filling defects. These defects change the position or disappear after additional swallows and therefore are easily distinguished from pathologic conditions.

3.2. Normal Function

In the upright position, liquids are transported from the mouth to the stomach primarily by gravity. Peristalsis plays almost no role. For this reason, testing of esophageal motility must be performed in the recumbent position to eliminate the effects of gravity. Temperature, viscosity, and volume of the liquid bolus may alter normal peristalsis, so these factors must be controlled when testing esophageal function. In addition, boluses must be spaced out to avoid the effect of deglutitive inhibition. Deglutitive inhibition is a

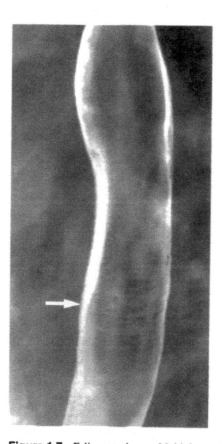

Figure 1.7 Feline esophagus. Multiple evenly spaced transverse folds are seen in the esophageal body (arrow). (With permission from Mayo Foundation, Johnson CD. Alimentary Tract Imaging: A Teaching File. Mosby-Yearbook, 1993.)

normal physiologic response to rapid drinking of liquids. To permit rapid ingestion of large amounts of liquids, the esophageal body relaxes as it fills following successive swallows. No peristaltic contraction occurs until after the final swallow, which clears remaining bolus from the esophageal body. During the barium exam if the patient swallows more than once in rapid succession, then the failure of peristalsis as a result of this normal physiologic reflex may be interpreted as abnormal function. With a large field of view image intensifier additional unintended swallows can be suspected by observing esophageal shortening due to contraction of the longitudinal muscles, which accompanies normal swallowing.

In the recumbent position barium bolus is transported by peristaltic contractions that cause the walls of the esophagus to oppose as the wave progresses down the esophagus and push the bolus toward the stomach. Not every swallow is accompanied by effective transport of barium bolus. Incomplete clearance is commonly seen in the middle third of the esophagus where velocity and amplitude of the peristaltic contraction is lowest. Using the technique described earlier complete clearance of bolus should occur in three out of five swallows (2). Unlike liquids, solid bolus transport requires peristalsis to move it into the stomach, even in the upright position. Normal transport of solid bolus (e.g., standard hamburger bolus) in the upright position may require up to four swallows for complete clearance (17).

Rapid swallowing of barium in the recumbent position (full-column technique) produces maximal physiologic distension of the esophageal body. The diameter of maximally distended esophagus provides a crude estimate of esophageal compliance. The maximum esophageal diameter (MED) is determined by measuring the largest diameter of the distended esophagus in the area between the aortic arch and the esophageal ampulla (measured on the three-on-one full-column films). In normal subjects this measurement is between 20 and 33 mm. Larger MEDs tend to occur in patients with hypomotility disorders (e.g., NEMD, achalasia, and scleroderma), which are associated with increased esophageal compliance. An abnormally small diameter may occur in patients who are unable to drink fast enough to maximally distend the esophagus. This can be suspected if one sees a discontinuous column of barium on the full-column films. Small diameters may also be seen in patients with abnormally decreased esophageal compliance due to stiffening of the wall as a result of inflammatory infiltrate or fibrosis.

4. HIATAL HERNIAS

Detection and characterization of hiatal hernias is important for a number of reasons. If the hernia is large (>5 cm in length), such as an intrathoracic stomach, the hernia is likely to be symptomatic. Torsion of large hernias may lead to life-threatening gastric ischemia (18). In addition, the surgical approach for the repair of a hernia is influenced by the type, size, and reducibility of the hernia. Large hernias that are difficult to reduce laparoscopically may result in tension on the repair when reduced leading to recurrence. Hernias of such size should probably be approached by a thoracic approach if it appears that they cannot be reduced without tension (19). Lastly, evidence suggests that given the same lower esophageal sphincter (LES) dysfunction, the severity of GERD is proportional to the size of the hernia (20).

The most common hiatal hernias are classified into four types based on the relationship of the GEJ and gastric fundus to the diaphragmatic hiatus (Fig. 1.8). Type 1 is the most common (~80%) and consists of symmetrical herniation of the GEJ and a variable portion of the stomach into the chest (Fig. 1.9). Type 2 hernias (<5%), also known as paraesophageal hernias, occur when the GEJ remains fixed at or below the hiatus and a

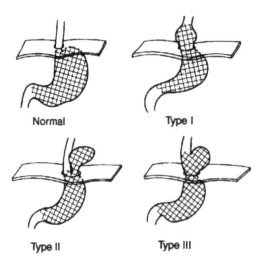

Figure 1.8 Hernia types. (Reprinted with permission from Jamieson GG, Duranceau A. Gastroesophageal Reflux. Elsevier, 1988:24.)

portion of stomach herniates through the hiatus (usually located left anterior) (Fig. 1.10). Pure Type 2 hernias are uncommon. Type 3 hernias (~15%) probably evolve from smaller Type 1 hernias and consist of a paraesophageal gastric component as well as upward displacement of the GEJ (Fig. 1.11). An intrathoracic stomach (Fig. 1.12) represents a severe

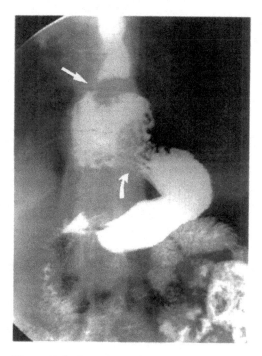

Figure 1.9 Type 1 hiatal hernia. Symmetrical hernia sac with GEJ (tubulovestibular junction) (straight arrow) well above the hiatus (curved arrow).

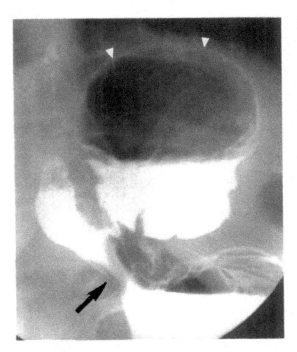

Figure 1.10   Type 2 hiatal hernia. GEJ remains below the hiatus (arrow) with large paraesopha-geal hernia (arrowheads).

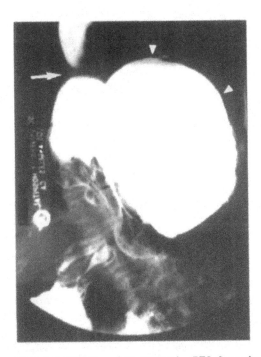

Figure 1.11   Type 3 hiatal hernia. GEJ above the hiatus and paraesophageal component.

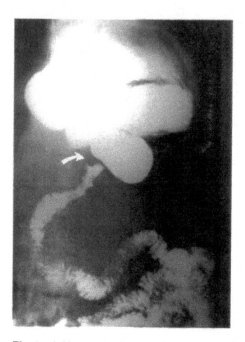

Figure 1.12   Large intrathoracic stomach. Pylorus at the level of the esophageal hiatus (arrow).

Type 3 hernia. The rare Type 4 hernia contains other organs, such as mesentery, liver, colon, etc., which herniate into the chest through a markedly enlarged hiatus.

Displacement of the GEJ above the esophageal hiatus constitutes a sliding hernia (Type 1) or mixed (Type 3) hernia. Small hernias (<2 cm) are probably not clinically important, so we need not worry about detecting them. It is also important to understand that the radiographically defined GEJ does not necessarily correspond to the endo-scopically or manometrically defined GEJ, and therefore, estimated hernia size will vary depending upon how it is measured. These comments aside, to detect hiatal hernias radiographically one must be able to locate both the GEJ and the esophageal hiatus. If the GEJ is >2 cm above the hiatus, a sliding hernia or mixed hernia exists.

There are several ways to radiographically define the GEJ. If a mucosal ring is visible it accurately defines the transition from squamous epithelium of the esophagus to columnar epithelium of the stomach. Otherwise, the tubulovestibular junction marks the lower end of the esophagus and the proximal stomach. Occasionally, gastric rugal folds are visible in the herniated portion of the stomach. This method is found to be the most difficult because rugal folds may resemble esophageal folds radiographically. Because the motor activity of the esophagus and stomach is different (peristaltic activity in the esophagus vs. tonic activity in the gastric fundus) the point at which peristalsis ends or slows, as observed fluoroscopically, indicates the functional transition point from the esophagus into the stomach.

The esophageal hiatus is more easily defined. Because the esophageal hiatus is bound by portions of the muscular diaphragm, that contracts during inspiration, the point of maximum narrowing of the esophagus during inspiration marks the position of the esophageal hiatus (Fig. 1.13). Now with both the GEJ and hiatus localized one can measure and characterize the hiatal hernia.

In patients undergoing antireflux surgery, an estimate of the chances of successfully reducing a hiatal hernia surgically without tension is an important consideration when

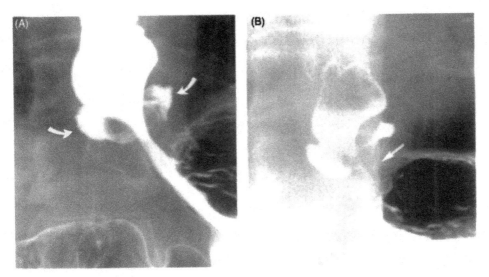

Figure 1.13 Position of esophageal hiatus. (A) During quiet respiration position of diaphragmatic hiatus is unclear. (B) Contraction of the diaphragm during deep inspiration produces narrowing of the esophagus at the level of the hiatus (straight arrow). Contrast fills the "wings" of the disrupted wrap (curved arrows).

planning the surgical approach. If one fails to reduce the hernia without tension surgical failure may result. A shortened esophagus (either congenital or acquired due to fibrosis and scarring) can lead to surgical failure if not recognized preoperatively (21). A sign that suggests a shortened esophagus is irreducibility of the hiatal hernia during barium exam. Estimation of reducibility can be made by comparing the size of the hiatal hernia on recumbent films with that on erect films. In the erect position, with the stomach filled with barium, the weight of the stomach tends to reduce the hernia into the abdomen. If the hernia does not reduce in the upright position the surgeons should be concerned that they will not be able to reduce it surgically without tension and may need to consider a different surgical approach. Likewise, large hernias (>5 cm) may be difficult to reduce laparoscopically without increased risk of surgical failure.

The shape of the hiatal hernia may also suggest a shortened esophagus. A hernia with rounded shoulders (resembling a cabernet bottle) (Fig. 1.14) is not usually associated with a shortened esophagus and will usually reduce surgically. On the other hand, a hernia with tapered elongated shoulders superiorly (resembling a chardonnay bottle) (Fig. 1.15) is frequently accompanied by scarring and may not reduce without tension.

5. GERD

Barium studies and GER have been linked together since GERD was first described. Early studies suggested that the barium exam was indeed a sensitive test for diagnosis of GERD. Unfortunately, these studies compared barium exams with the presence of heartburn or esophagitis, as an indication of reflux disease. We now know that heartburn is a nonspecific symptom and occurs in <70% of patients with positive ambulatory pH testing (22). Esophagitis is even less sensitive for GERD and only occurs in approximately

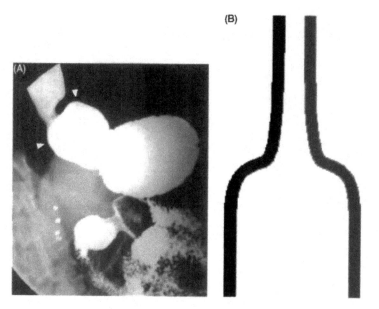

Figure 1.14   Normal esophageal length—"cabernet"-shaped hiatal hernia. (A) Type 1 hiatal hernia with rounded shoulders resembling shoulders of a cabernet wine bottle (B) suggesting normal esophageal length.

half of patients with reflux disease (23). Several recent studies compared the presence of GER on barium swallows with results of ambulatory pH monitoring (24–28). Ambulatory pH testing is accepted as a highly accurate test for the presence of GER. The results of these studies vary but support the view that barium swallows are relatively insensitive

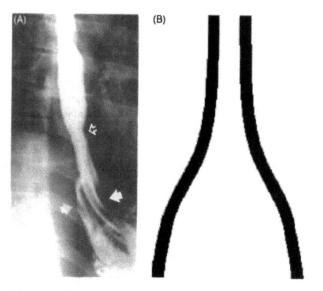

Figure 1.15   Shortened esophagus—"chardonnay"-shaped hiatal hernia. (A) Hiatal hernia with tapered shoulders (closed arrows) and associated irregular stricture (open arrow) resembling a (B) chardonnay wine bottle.

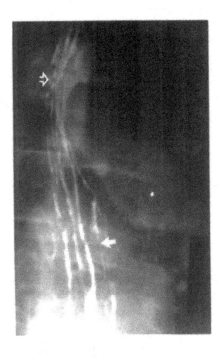

Figure 1.16 Acute reflux esophagitis. Mucosal relief images showing thickened (closed arrow) discontinous (open arrow) folds in the distal esophagus.

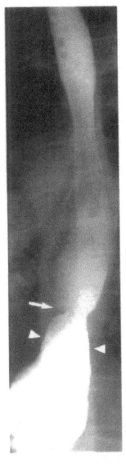

Figure 1.17 Advanced scleroderma of the esophagus. Tapered shoulders of hiatal hernia (arrowheads) indicate esophageal shortening ("chardonnay-shaped" hernia) with stricture at GEJ (arrow). Marked stasis of contrast in esophageal body from severe hypomotility.

and nonspecific in detecting GER. As a screening test the barium exam does not have a role in the detection of GER, but is helpful in evaluating patients for a number of other reasons.

One of the most important reasons to perform barium studies in GERD is to exclude other conditions that may mimic GERD. As mentioned earlier, heartburn and regurgitation are very nonspecific symptoms and are seen in a variety of esophageal diseases. For example, 40% of patients with achalasia complain of heartburn. Experience at USC suggests that up to 7% of patients with typical symptoms of GERD have a primary motility disorder instead, usually achalasia. As therapy for these two conditions is very different it is important to make this distinction prior to treatment.

Mucosal diseases can be diagnosed with barium studies; however, endoscopy is far more sensitive, especially in reflux esophagitis and Barrett's esophagus. Reflux esophagitis can be healed or greatly improved with proton pump inhibitors reducing the degree of severity seen endoscopically. Untreated, severe esophagitis is uncommonly seen in our practice. Although barium exams are relatively sensitive in detecting severe esophagitis (Fig. 1.16) mild disease usually goes undetected (29). Esophageal scarring, accompanying injury from severe GERD, produces characteristic prominent transverse ridges in the distal esophagus and is readily diagnosed with barium exams.

There are a number of additional indications for performance of a barium swallow in GERD patients. Diagnosis of strictures or motility disorders in the dysphagic GERD patient (Fig. 1.17), evaluation of recurrent symptoms in patients with a history of previous antireflux surgery (Fig. 1.18), and detection of GERD-associated abnormalities (Figs. 1.19 and 1.20) are important reasons to perform the study.

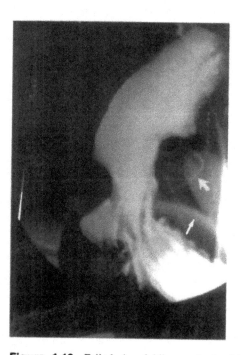

Figure 1.18 Failed Angelchik prosthesis. Metallic ring representing Angelchik prosthesis (large arrow) visible above diaphragm (small arrow).

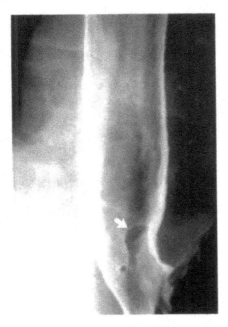

Figure 1.19 Inflammatory pseudopolyp in GERD. Thickened gastric fold producing club-shaped polypoid filling defect (arrow) at GEJ.

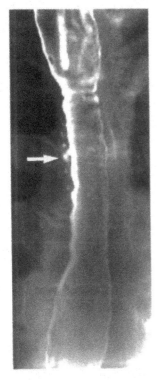

Figure 1.20 Intramural pseudodiverticulosis. Numerous small outpouchings (arrow) due to dilated submucous glands, probably the result of chronic inflammation. (With permission from Mayo Foundation, Johnson CD. Alimentary Tract Imaging: A Teaching File. Mosby-Yearbook, 1993.)

6. SEGMENTAL NARROWING

The three most common causes of dysphagia are cancer, benign stricture, and motility disorders. A careful clinical history will frequently provide clues to narrow the differential diagnosis. Dysphagia to solid foods is more common in mechanical narrowing, such as cancer or benign strictures, whereas difficulty with both solids and liquids more likely indicates a motility disorder. Bariums studies are useful for the evaluation of all causes of dysphagia—both structural narrowing and abnormal motility. In the detection of esophageal carcinoma, the barium swallow has been shown to be very sensitive (30). Unfortunately, patients with esophageal cancer who present with dysphagia usually have advanced disease and the chance for curative therapy is small. Barium studies are superior to endoscopy in detecting benign causes of segmental narrowing (14). The exam also provides information regarding motility and may provide useful information prior to endoscopy. This makes it an attractive screening test for dysphagic patients.

The ability to detect strictures requires proper technique. As discussed earlier, to optimize detection of structural narrowing, full-column films with maximal filling of the esophagus in the prone oblique position are necessary. With the esophagus maximally distended, areas of narrowing become apparent. In general, areas of segmental narrowing >20 mm seldom cause symptoms. On the other hand, narrowing <13–15 mm is almost always associated with symptoms (31) (Fig. 1.21). It is therefore necessary to measure the diameter of areas of segmental narrowing not only to determine clinical significance but also to provide a baseline measurement prior to therapeutic dilatation.

A variety of benign conditions cause mechanical narrowing in the esophagus. Webs occur in the proximal cervical esophagus, usually on the anterior wall, and appear as a shelf-like membrane (Fig. 1.22) (32). These must be differentiated from a

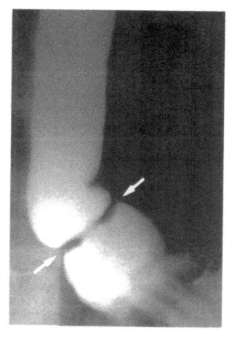

Figure 1.21   Mucosal ring. Concentric shelf-like narrowing characteristic of mucosal ring.

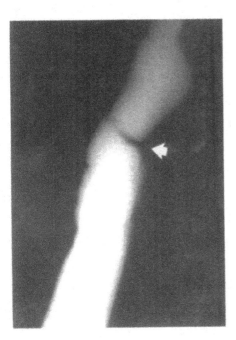

Figure 1.22 Esophageal web. Anterior shelf-like defect in cervical esophagus (arrowhead).

normal postcricoid impression that is usually more broad-based and does not produce appreciable narrowing. Because webs are fragile, symptoms are commonly cured by disruption of the webs during passage of an endoscope and therefore escape radiologic diagnosis.

Zenker's diverticula (Fig. 1.23) are pulsion-type diverticula that occur above the cricopharyngeus through a congenital defect in the wall of the pharynx known as Killian's dehiscence. They are frequently associated with cervical dysphagia and may be be associated with airway penetration. Spontaneous regurgitation of undigested food from the diverticulum is a classic symptom.

Cricopharyngeal bars (Fig. 1.24) (also called cricopharyngeal achalasia) are commonly seen during barium studies, especially in the elderly. Pathologically, they are the result of degeneration of the striated muscle that alters the compliance and may produce pharyngeal outlet obstruction. Assigning the cause of the patient's dysphagia to a cricopharyngeal bar should be done with caution. Bars are very common but uncommonly are associated with dysphagia. Large bars (producing >50% narrowing of the distended pharynx) and those which are constant throughout the swallow are more likely to be symptomatic than small transient defects (33,34).

Causes of high strictures (Fig. 1.25) include Barrett's strictures, caustic ingestion, radiation injury, pill injury, eosinophilic esophagitis, and skin disease-associated strictures. Long strictures are commonly seen with radiation-induced injury and lye ingestion. In these cases the etiology will be obvious from the clinical history. Barrett's strictures occur at the proximal end of the columnar-lined esophagus and may have associated reticular mucosal pattern and other GERD-associated changes such as scarring, esophageal shortening, and hiatal hernia. Pill strictures usually occur as a result of mucosal irritation at the site where the pill lodges—usually at the level of the aortic arch or left main bronchus.

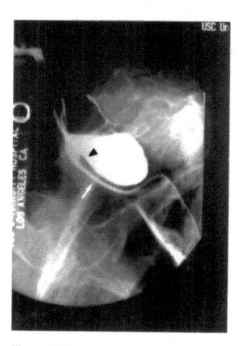

Figure 1.23 Zenker's diverticulum. Large Zenker's diverticulum arising just above the cricopharyngeus (black arrowhead). Esophageal lumen being displaced by diverticulum (arrow).

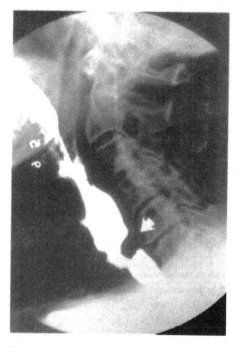

Figure 1.24 Cricopharyngeal bar. Posterior defect in cervical esophagus usually at C5–6
level (arrow). With the esophagus maximally distended, bar produces ~70% narrowing of the lumen.

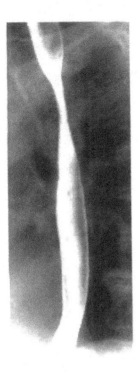

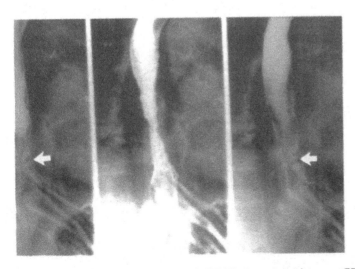

Figure 1.25 Pill stricture. Forty-five-year-old female with solid food dysphagia and history of chronic NSAID use for arthritis.

Areas of segmental narrowing in the distal esophagus are caused by mucosal rings and inflammatory strictures. By far, the most common stricture in the distal esophagus is associated with GERD (Fig. 1.26). These strictures are located near the GEJ and are usually associated with hiatal hernias. They are often eccentric and may have an irregular

Figure 1.26 Scarring and stricture in GERD. Irregular stricture at GEJ with transverse scarring typical of GERD related injury (arrows).

contour or consist of multiple transverse folds. They may be gradually tapered or have an abrupt transition. Their appearance is usually sufficiently characteristic to differentiate them from malignant strictures (Fig. 1.27). Strictures associated with scleroderma, Zollinger–Ellison, and prolonged NG intubation have a similar pathogenesis and appearance.

An uncommon but important cause of dysphagia in young patients is the small caliber esophagus. These patients have long-standing complaints of dysphagia to solid foods. The cause of their dysphagia usually goes undetected for years. Endoscopy is usually normal or shows areas of ring-like narrowing. Characteristically the esophagus has a normal contour but is narrowed uniformly throughout its length. Diagnosis is based on recognition of a MED of <20 mm. In the majority of cases, esophageal biopsies suggest eosinophilic esophagitis. Those with positive biopsies are likely to respond to treatment with topical steroids.

Dysphagia lusoria is a rare cause of dysphagia and occurs as a result of vascular rings, usually an aberrant origin of the left subclavian artery (Fig. 1.28).

7. MOTILITY DISORDERS

7.1. Achalasia

Achalasia is the most common primary esophageal motility disorder. It is characterized by diminished peristalsis in the esophageal body and abnormal LES function, which produces

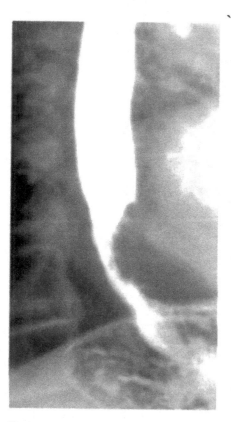

Figure 1.27 Esophageal cancer. Shelf-like appearance at the upper end. With irregular edge.

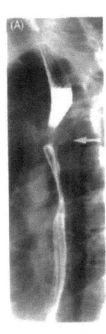
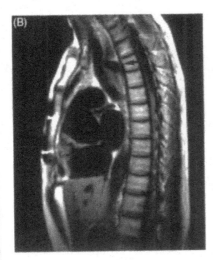

Figure 1.28 Dysphagia lusoria due to aberrant right subclavian artery. (A) Lateral view barium swallow shows posterior defect at aortic arch level (arrow). (B) Sagittal MR or chest demonstrates aberrant right subclavian artery coursing behind esophagus (arrow).

esophageal outlet obstruction. In its classic form it is easily diagnosed with a barium swallow (Fig. 1.29). Findings include a flaccid, dilated esophageal body that fails to empty in the upright position. The "bird's beak" deformity (Fig. 1.30) described in achalasia is the result of a hypertensive LES, which produces esophageal outlet obstruction.

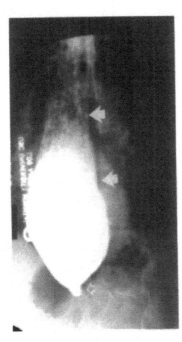

Figure 1.29 Classic achalasia. Debris and barium retained in massive dilated esophagus (closed arrows) with tapered narrowing of distal esophagus (open arrow).

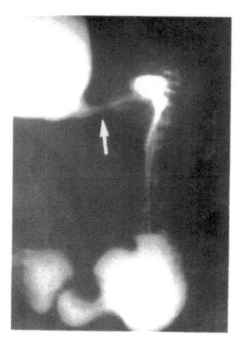

Figure 1.30   Classic achalasia with bird's beak deformity of distal esophagus (arrow).

In severe cases, the esophagus becomes massively dilated, tortuous, and elongated (sigmoid esophagus) with dependent areas that prevent adequate drainage in the upright position (Fig. 1.31). This condition is important to recognize on a barium study because therapeutic dilatation or myotomy may be less effective in promoting esophageal emptying.

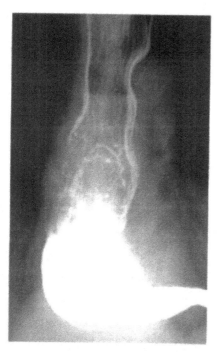

Figure 1.31   Achalasia. Tortuous, elongated "sigmoid" esophagus drains poor in the upright position. As a result, therapeutic drainage procedures may not be successful.

Not uncommonly, classic findings of achalasia may not be present, especially in mild cases. In these cases, the esophageal body may be only mildly dilated and empties normally in the upright position. The only clue to the diagnosis may be ineffective or disordered peristalsis. Absence of outflow obstruction is attributed to the fact that there is little or no elevation of the LES resting pressure, therefore, the hydrostatic pressure of the barium column easily overcomes the outflow resistance. Without manometry these patients may be misdiagnosed as ineffective esophageal motility (IEM) or other hypomotility disorders. It is important to recognize these patients and refer them for manometry because they are likely to benefit from therapeutic drainage procedures.

In a minority of patients with achalasia, an increase in tertiary contractions will be seen instead of a flaccid esophageal body. This uncommon variant is called vigorous achalasia (Fig. 1.32). Associated findings may include moderate dilatation of the esophageal body and incomplete emptying in the upright position. Differentiation from other spastic disorders may be difficult especially if signs of esophageal outlet obstruction are absent.

Patients with pseudoachalasia may have an identical appearance with classic achalasia. In some cases of pseudoachalasia, when compared with classic achalasia, the length of the distal esophageal narrowing is longer and the esophagus is less dilated (35). The etiology of pseudoachalasia is an invasive malignancy arising in the region of the GEJ (Fig. 1.33). Tumor invasion of the myenteric plexus may disturb esophageal innervation and cause motor abnormalities producing a clinical picture identical to that of achalasia. A short clinical history and advanced age of the patient provide clues to the diagnosis especially in patients with typical radiographic findings of achalasia.

Conventional treatment for achalasia consists of therapeutic dilatation or distal esophageal myotomy. Esophageal perforation is an unusual complication following balloon dilatation. If there is a clinical suspicion of perforation, a contrast study is indicated. A small number of perforations may not be visible with a contrast swallow.

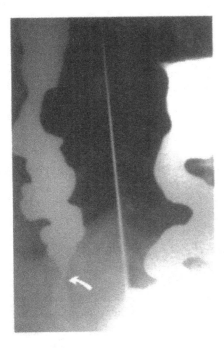

Figure 1.32 Vigorous achalasia. Dilated esophageal body with prominent tertiary contractions and tapered narrowing at GEJ (curved arrow).

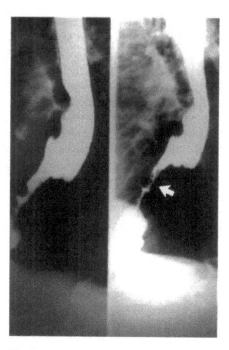

Figure 1.33   Pseudoachalasia. Dilated esophageal body with irregular narrowing of GEJ (arrow) due to adenocarcinoma. Irregular, eccentric narrowing differentiates this from classic achalasia.

If there is a strong clinical suspicion of perforation, CT scanning may demonstrate extravasation of contrast, pneumomediastinum, or pneumothorax. Following Heller myotomy, a typical pseudodiverticulum deformity of the distal esophagus may be seen (Fig. 1.34).

The esophagus is affected in 80% of patients with scleroderma. This degenerative disorder of the smooth muscle causes decreased amplitude of contractions in the distal two-thirds of the esophagus. In addition, involvement of the smooth muscle of the LES results in loss of antireflux barrier. Ineffective peristalsis promotes injury to the esophagus as a result of poor esophageal clearance of refluxate. Radiographically, these patients have findings of severe reflux disease—hernias, shortened esophagus, strictures, Barrett's, etc. In mild disease, only the signs of poor esophageal body function are seen, namely stasis and mild dilatation of the esophageal body. Similar but less severe changes are seen in other collagen diseases.

Spastic disorders of the esophagus include diffuse esophageal spasm, nutcracker esophagus, hypertensive LES, and vigorous achalasia. Barium swallows are normal in nutcracker esophagus and hypertensive LES. Classic findings in patients with diffuse esophageal spasm include the "corkscrew" and "rosary-bead" esophagus (Fig. 1.35). Unfortunately, characteristic findings occur in a minority of patients with this uncommon disease.

Pulsion diverticula (Fig. 1.36) are associated with spastic disorders of the esophagus (36). A narrow neck and location in the distal third of the esophagus distinguish them from traction diverticula (Fig. 1.37) which are due to paraesophageal inflammatory scarring secondary to granulomatous mediastinal adenitis. These diverticula have broad-based neck and appear as if "pulled" from the esophageal wall.

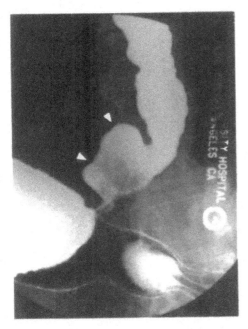

Figure 1.34 Status post Heller myotomy deformity. Eccentric broad-based diverticular-like contrast collection (arrowheads) from previous myotomy.

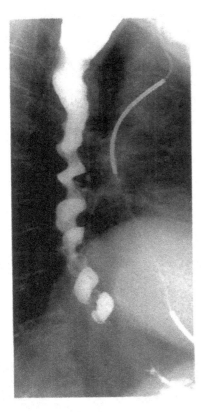

Figure 1.35 Diffuse esophageal spasm associated with "corkscrew" esophagus.

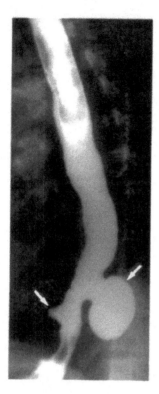

Figure 1.36 Pulsion diverticula. One large and one small pulsion diverticula (arrows) seen in the distal esophagus in these patients with abnormal esophageal motility diagnosed by manometry.

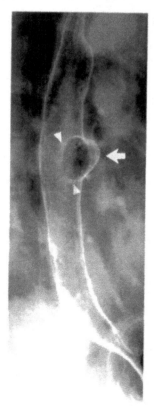

Figure 1.37 Traction diverticulum. Mid-esophageal location (arrow) and wide neck of the diverticulum (arrowheads) are characteristic of traction diverticulum.

8. POSTOPERATIVE IMAGING

Barium studies are commonly performed in the immediate postoperative period to exclude early complications such as anastomotic leak. Early detection of leaks is important to avoid septic complications. Barium, with its superior radiodensity, would seem to be the contrast media of choice, however, evidence suggests that extravasated barium may produce an inflammatory response. Water-soluble contrast, on the other hand, is rapidly absorbed, should extravasation occur, but may produce severe pulmonary edema if aspirated. Therefore, the choice of contrast media to use should be considered carefully (37). Prior to the exam the patients should be evaluated clinically to assess their ability to safely swallow oral contrast without aspirating. A higher risk of aspiration exists in the recumbent position so if the patient is unable to stand one should consider postponing the study until the patient is able to do so. If the patient seems lethargic or otherwise unable to cooperate, the use of barium rather than water-soluble contrast should be considered. The risk of complications from aspiration of water-soluble contrast usually outweighs that from extravasation of barium. Our technique in evaluating patients in the early postoperative period is summarized in Fig. 1.38.

Anastomotic leaks occur in 6–26% of patients undergoing esophagectomy (38). Most leaks occur proximally at the esophagogastric anastamosis (or esophagocolic anastamosis in the case of a colon interpositions) because of its vulnerability to ischemia. Careful examination with water-soluble contrast or barium will detect most leaks and provide an estimate of the size of the leak. In those cases in which clinical suspicion is high, even though the contrast study may be negative, CT scanning with oral and IV contrast may be helpful in demonstrating a leak as well as associated fluid collections (38). If necessary, percutaneous CT-guided drainage can be performed at the same time.

Following fundoplication a barium swallow may be requested to assess position and configuration of the wrap, to provide a baseline exam and to assess esophageal emptying. Barium can be used in this circumstance because there is little risk of perforation unless the enteric lumen has been violated during surgery. The normal Nissen fundoplication appears as a rounded soft tissue density in the fundus of the stomach with a narrowed esophageal lumen traversing the center of the wrap (Fig. 1.39). The central esophageal channel should be straight or curved gently. An improperly constructed fundoplication may be acutely angulated as a result of tension on the wrap. As a result of postoperative swelling/hematoma there is diminished or disordered motility and delayed emptying of the distal esophageal body. Immediately after surgery, the soft issue density representing the wrap is approximately the size of a lemon. Over the following months and years the wrap becomes oval-shaped and decreases to about the size of a small plum.

The radiographic appearance of a partial fundoplication is similar to a complete fundoplication (i.e., Nissen), except that the fundal soft tissue mass is smaller and

Radiographic evaluation after esophageal surgery
• Perform in upright position
• Videotape in multiple projections
• Start with H$_2$O soluble or barium? Is patient likely to aspirate?
• Use enough volume to exclude leak
• Don't over-diagnose anastamotic narrowing

Figure 1.38 Postoperative barium swallow technique.

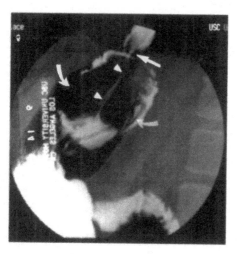

Figure 1.39 Normal Nissen fundoplication. Soft tissue produced by wrap visible in gastric fundus (curved arrows) with central luminal narrowing (arrowheads). There is no gastric cardia above wrap, therefore, no evidence of "slipped Nissen." Position of hiatus visible (straight arrow) above gastric cardia, therefore, no hiatal hernia.

lumen of the esophagus is eccentrically positioned within the wrap. As with a Nissen fundoplication the wrap should be located below the diaphragm and no hiatal hernia should be seen. Figure 1.40 shows the appearance of an esophageal lengthening procedure (Collis gastroplasty), which is sometimes used in a shortened esophagus, and is usually accompanied by a partial fundoplication.

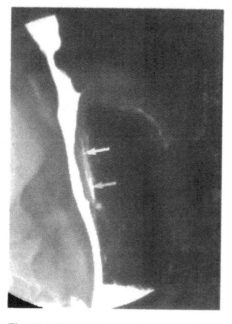

Figure 1.40 Collis gastroplasty with Belsey Mark IV fundoplication. Staple line (arrows) separates lengthened esophagus from gastric fundus.

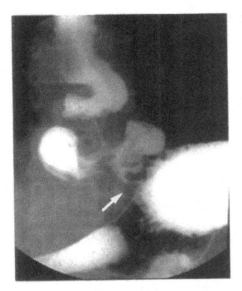

Figure 1.41 Disrupted Nissen fundoplication. Bizarre "clover leaf" shaped hiatal hernia visible above the hiatus (arrow).

In a minority of patients structural failure of the fundoplication can produce recurrent or new symptoms. Disruption of the wrap, intrathoracic migration of the wrap or malposition of the fundoplication in the stomach rather than the GEJ (so-called slipped Nissen) may occur. The presence of a hiatal hernia (Fig. 1.41) or abundant contrast in the "wings" of the wrap indicates partial or complete disruption. Subtle disruptions may be difficult to detect unless proper technique is used (Fig. 1.42). Air-contrast

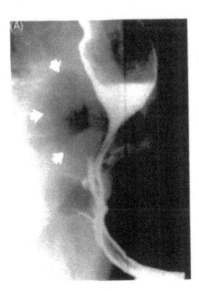
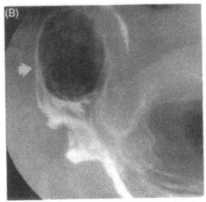

Figure 1.42 Importance of technique in demonstrating recurrent hiatal hernia after failed fundoplication. (A) Air in paraesophageal hernia (arrows) barely visible on this upright film. (B) After the patient is placed supine and then upright, the hernia becomes obvious (arrow) on this air-contrast film.

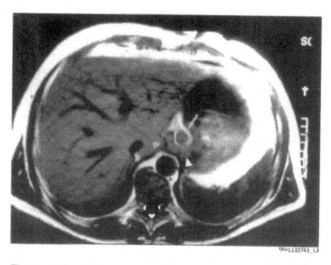

Figure 1.43 MR appearance of intact Nissen fundoplication. "Hot-dog-in-a-bun" configuration of intact wrap. Esophagus ("hot dog," arrow) passing through the center of the wrap ("bun," arrowheads).

technique should be performed. After the patients have been given gas crystals and high-density barium they should be placed in the supine position to fill the fundus. The presence of barium in a hernia sac above the hiatus or in the "wings" of the fundoplication will indicate disruption. If none is seen the patient should be brought upright and the area of fundus again examined. In this position, air may bubble up though a narrow opening into a hernia and become visible above the diaphragm.

Frequently, the cause of recurrent symptoms following antireflux surgery is not clear. Endoscopy, barium studies, and ambulatory testing may be negative or contradictory. MR imaging may be helpful in evaluating these patients. MR has the advantage of multiplanar depiction of anatomy and superior soft tissue discrimination.

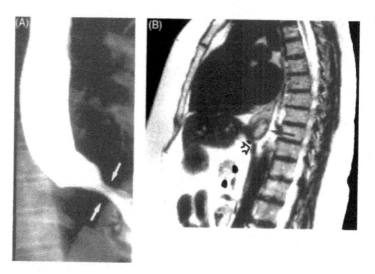

Figure 1.44 Malpositioned Nissen. Fifty-year-old female with dysphagia and chest pain following fundoplication. (A) Barium swallow shows narrowing (arrows) of distal esophagus. (B) Sagittal MR scan demonstrates fundoplication (arrow) above the diaphragm (open arrow).

Nissen fundoplications have a characteristic MR appearance as illustrated in Fig. 1.43. Our preliminary experience suggests that MR is capable of detecting wrap disruption, malposition, and recurrent hernia. Its usefulness is illustrated in Fig. 1.44.

REFERENCES

1. Hewson EG et al. Manometry and radiology. Complementary studies in the assessment of esophageal motility disorders. Gastroenterology 1990; 98(3):626–632.
2. Fuller L et al. Abnormal esophageal body function: radiographic–manometric correlation. Am Surg 1999; 65(10):911–914.
3. Dodds WJ, Logemann JA, Stewart ET. Radiologic assessment of abnormal oral and pharyngeal phases of swallowing. Am J Roentgenol 1990; 154(5):965–974.
4. Dodds WJ, Stewart ET, Logemann JA. Physiology and radiology of the normal oral and pharyngeal phases of swallowing. Am J Roentgenol 1990; 154(5):953–963.
5. Anbari MM et al. Delayed leaks and fistulas after esophagogastrectomy: radiologic evaluation. Am J Roentgenol 1993; 160(6):1217–1220.
6. Block M et al. Improvement in staging of esophageal cancer with the addition of positron emission tomography. Ann Thorac Surg 1997; 64:770–777.
7. Flamen P et al. The utility of positron emission tomography for the diagnosis and staging of recurrent esophageal cancer. J Thorac Cardiovasc Surg 2000; 120:1085–1092.
8. Himeno S et al. Evaluation of esophageal cancer by positron emission tomography. Jpn J Clin Oncol 2002; 32:340–346.
9. Luketich J et al. Role of positron emission tomography in staging esophageal cancer. Ann Thorac Surg 1997; 64:765–769.
10. Halpert RD, Spickler E, Feczko PJ. Dysphagia in patients with gastric cancer and a normal esophagram. Radiology 1985; 154(3):589–591.
11. Wilcox CM, Alexander LN, Clark WS. Localization of an obstructing esophageal lesion. Is the patient accurate? Dig Dis Sci 1995; 40(10):2192–2196.
12. Brady AP et al. Premature contraction of the cricopharyngeus: a new sign of gastroesophageal reflux disease. Abdom Imaging 1995; 20(3):225–229.
13. Ekberg O, Lindgren S. Gastroesophageal reflux and pharyngeal function. Acta Radiologica: Diagnosis 1986; 27(4):421–423.
14. Ott DJ et al. Radiographic and endoscopic sensitivity in detecting lower esophageal mucosal ring. Am J Roentgenol 1986; 147(2):261–265.
15. Lin S et al. The phrenic ampulla: distal esophagus or potential hiatal hernia? Am J Physiol 1995; 268(2 Pt 1):G320–G327.
16. Rencken IO et al. Ringed esophagus (feline esophagus) in childhood. Pediatr Radiol 1997; 27(9):773–775.
17. Pouderoux P et al. Esophageal solid bolus transit: studies using concurrent videofluoroscopy and manometry. Am J Gastroenterol 1999; 94(6):1457–1463.
18. Ellis FH. Esophageal hiatal hernia. N Engl J Med 1972; 287(13):646–649.
19. Hashemi M et al. Laparoscopic repair of large type III hiatal hernia: objective followup reveals high recurrence rate. J Am Coll Surg 2000; 190(5):553–560; discussion 560–561.
20. Sloan S, Rademaker AW, Kahrilas PJ. Determinants of gastroesophageal junction incompetence: hiatal hernia, lower esophageal sphincter, or both? (comment). Ann Intern Med 1992; 117(12):977–982.
21. Gastal OL et al. Short esophagus: analysis of predictors and clinical implications. Arch Surg 1999; 134(6):633–636; discussion 637–638.
22. Tefera L et al. Can the combination of symptoms and endoscopy confirm the presence of gastroesophageal reflux disease? Am Surg 1997; 63(10):933–936.
23. Locke GR III. Natural history of nonerosive reflux disease. Is all gastroesophageal reflux disease the same? What is the evidence? (Review) (22 refs). Gastroenterol Clin North America 2002; 31(suppl 4):S59–S66.

24. Chen MY et al. Gastroesophageal reflux disease: correlation of esophageal pH testing and radiographic findings. Radiology 1992; 185(2):483–486.

25. Fransson SG et al. Radiologic diagnosis of gastro-oesophageal reflux by means of graded abdominal compression. Acta Radiol 1988; 29(1):45–48.

26. Johnston BT et al. Comparison of barium radiology with esophageal pH monitoring in the diagnosis of gastroesophageal reflux disease. Am J Gastroenterol 1996; 91(6):1181–1185.

27. Sellar RJ, De Caestecker JS, Heading RC. Barium radiology: a sensitive test for gastro-oesophageal reflux. Clin Radiol 1987; 38(3):303–307.

28. Thompson JK, Koehler RE, Richter JE. Detection of gastroesophageal reflux: value of barium studies compared with 24-hr pH monitoring. Am J Roentgenol 1994; 162(3):621–626.

29. Ott DJ, Wu WC, Gelfand DW. Reflux esophagitis revisited: prospective analysis of radiologic accuracy. Gastrointest Radiol 1981; 6(1):1–7.

30. Levine MS et al. Carcinoma of the esophagus and esophagogastric junction: sensitivity of radiographic diagnosis. Am J Roentgenol 1997; 168(6):1423–1426.

31. Schatzki R, Gary J. Dysphagia due to a diaphragm-like localized narrowing in the lower esophagus ("lower esophageal ring"). Am J Roentgenol 1953; 70:911–922.

32. Clements JL Jr et al. Cervical esophageal webs—a roentgenanatomic correlation. Observations on the pharyngoesophagus. Am J Roentgenol Radium Ther Nucl Med 1974; 121(2):221–231.

33. Ekberg O, Nylander G. Cineradiography of the pharyngeal stage of deglutition in 250 patients with dysphagia. Br J Radiol 1982; 55(652):258–262.

34. Ekberg O, Nylander G. Cineradiography of the pharyngeal stage of deglutition in 150 individuals without dysphagia. Br J Radiol 1982; 55(652):253–257.

35. Woodfield CA et al. Diagnosis of primary versus secondary achalasia: reassessment of clinical and radiographic criteria. Am J Roentgenol 2000; 175(3):727–731.

36. Nehra D et al. Physiologic basis for the treatment of epiphrenic diverticulum. Ann Surg 2002; 235(3):346–354.

37. Levine MS. What is the best oral contrast material to use for the fluoroscopic diagnosis of esophageal rupture? (comment). Am J Roentgenol 1994; 162(5):1243.

38. Kim SH et al. Esophageal resection: indications, techniques, and radiologic assessment. (Review) (40 refs). Radiographics 2001; 21(5):1119–1137; discussion 1138–1140.

2
Esophageal Endoscopy

1. ENDOSCOPY

Endoscopic evaluation is necessary to confirm or establish a diagnosis in most esophageal disorders.

1.1. Specific Indications*

A. Upper abdominal symptoms that persist despite an appropriate trial of therapy;
B. Upper abdominal symptoms associated with other symptoms or signs suggesting serious organic disease (e.g., anorexia and weight loss) or in patients over 45 years of age;
C. Dysphagia or odynophagia;
D. Esophageal reflux symptoms, which are persistent or recurrent despite appropriate therapy;
E. Persistent vomiting of unknown cause;
F. Other diseases in which the presence of upper gastrointestinal (GI) pathology might modify other planned management. Examples include, patients who have a history of ulcer or GI bleeding, who are scheduled for organ transplantation, long-term anticoagulation, or chronic nonsteroidal anti-inflammatory drug therapy for arthritis and those with cancer of the head and neck;
G. Familial polyposis syndromes;
H. For confirmation and specific histologic diagnosis of radiologically demonstrated lesions such as
   1. suspected neoplastic lesion,
   2. gastric or esophageal ulcer,
   3. upper tract stricture or obstruction;
I. GI bleeding
   1. in patients with active or recent bleeding,
   2. for presumed chronic blood loss and for iron deficiency anemia when the clinical situation suggests an upper GI source or when colonoscopy is negative;
J. When sampling of tissue or fluid is indicated;

---

*American Society for Gastrointestinal Endoscopy. Consensus Statement. Gastrointest Endosc 2001; 52(6):831–837.

K.   In patients with suspected portal hypertension to document or treat esophageal varices;

L.   To assess acute injury after caustic ingestion;

M.   Treatment of bleeding lesions such as ulcers, tumors, and vascular abnormalities (e.g., electrocoagulation, heater probe, laser photocoagulation, or injection therapy);

N.   Banding or sclerotherapy of varices;

O.   Removal of foreign bodies;

P.   Removal of selected polypoid lesions;

Q.   Placement of feeding or drainage tubes (peroral, percutaneous endoscopic gastrostomy, and percutaneous endoscopic jejunostomy);

R.   Dilatation of stenotic lesions (e.g., with transendoscopic balloon dilators or dilation systems employing guide wires);

S.   Management of achalasia (e.g., botulinum toxin, balloon dilation);

T.   Palliative treatment of stenosing neoplasms (e.g., laser, multipolar electro-coagulation, and stent placement).

Esophago-gastro-duodenoscopy (EGD) is generally not indicated for evaluating the following.

A.   Symptoms that are considered functional in origin (there are exceptions in which an endoscopic examination may be done once to rule out organic disease, especially if symptoms are unresponsive to therapy);

B.   Metastatic adenocarcinoma of unknown primary site when the results will not alter management;

C.   Radiographic findings of
    1.   asymptomatic or uncomplicated sliding hiatal hernia,
    2.   uncomplicated duodenal ulcer which has responded to therapy,
    3.   deformed duodenal bulb when symptoms are absent or respond adequately to ulcer therapy.

Post gastric or colonic interposition. Unexplained fever or leucocytosis following gastric or colonic "pull-up" procedures may suggest graft necrosis. Early endoscopy, sometimes as early as 3 days after operation, may reveal patchy or even total graft necrosis and the need to remove the graft emergently.

1.2. Normal Anatomy

Evaluation of the esophagus starts with a good view of the vocal cords and ary-epiglottic folds. High gastroesophageal reflux is suspected in symptomatic patients who have inflammation of the posterior wall of the pharynx. The position of the cricopharyngeal sphincter is best assessed on the final withdrawal of the endoscope, and is noted by an encroachment on the lumen as the scope is withdrawn. When the endoscope enters the esophagus, the mucosa is whitish and fine vessels may be seen on the surface, especially at the lower end. The aortic arch causes a wall indentation usually at or beyond the 20 cm mark. The squamocolumnar junction is usually seen just proximal to the hiatus. It has a regular margin. When the patient is asked to sniff, the lumen of the esophagus narrows further. The gastroesophageal junction is identified at the top of the gastric mucosal folds that meet the tubular esophagus. When the endoscope enters the stomach there should be a minimal amount of clear secretion. The gastric mucosa is carefully inspected and its distensibility is noted. The endoscope is advanced into the duodenal bulb and

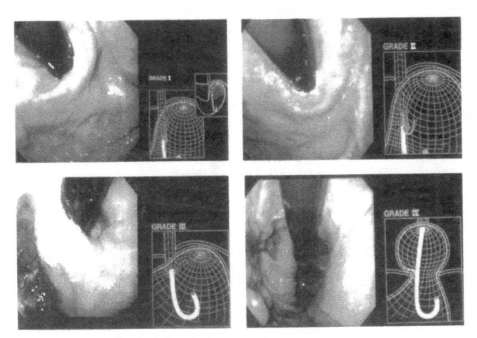

Figure 2.1 (**See color insert**) Hill's grading of the retroflexed view of the cardia. (With permission from Hill, Lucius D, Kozarek RA. The gastro-esophageal flap valve. J Clin Gastroenterol 1999; 28(3):194–197. *Grade I valve.* A ridge of tissue 3–4 cm long on the lesser curve is closely applied to the endoscope. *Grade II valve.* The ridge is less well defined than in Grade I and it opens occasionally with respiration but closes promptly. *Grade III valve.* The ridge is barely present and there is often failure to close around the endoscope. It is nearly always accompanied by a hiatal hernia and esophagitis. *Grade IV valve.* There is no muscular ridge. The gastroesophageal junction remains open all the time, and the squamous epithelium can often be seen from this retro-flexed position. A hiatal hernia is always present.

second part of the duodenum to exclude other pathologies. When the endoscope is retracted to the incisura level it is retroflexed to give a view of the gastroesophageal junction. The normal anatomy of the junction is noted and the stomach is insufflated to assess the competency of the lower esophageal sphincter and to grade the sphincter according to Hills' grading. The lesser and greater curvatures and the anterior and posterior aspects of the mucosa are systematically and carefully inspected for any abnor-malities. The stomach is deflated before retracting the instrument for a final viewing of the esophagus.

1.3. Biopsies

Biopsies from the retroflexed view of the squamocolumnar junction and the esophagus are recommended in patients who give a history of gastroesophageal reflux, especially if there is a history of GERD for more than 5 years so as to exclude Barrett's epithelium. Microscopic evidence of GERD may be present even in the absence of macroscopic esophagitis. It is routine in many clinics to biopsy the antrum for evidence of *Heucobacter pylori* infection. Any suspicious area should also be biopsied.

Gastroesophageal Valve Grade *Prevalence of acid exposure*

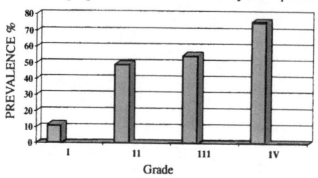

Figure 2.2 Correlation of Hill's grading of the gastroesophageal valve and the prevalence of acid exposure to the esophagus. (From Oberg S, Peters JH, DeMeester TR, Lord RV, Johannson J, Crookes PF, Bremner CG. Grading of the gastroesophageal valve in patients with symptoms of gastroesophageal reflux disease. Surg Endosc 1999; 12:1184–1188.)

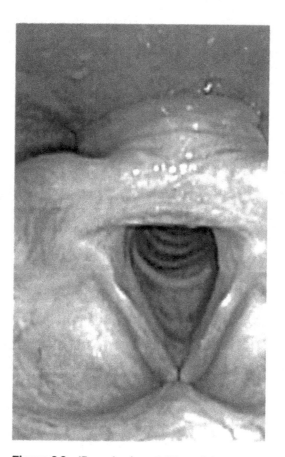

Figure 2.3 **(See color insert)** View of the normal vocal cords. High gastroesophageal reflux is suspected when posterior redness is seen. The cords are also inspected for movement.

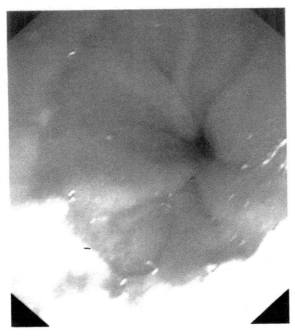

Figure 2.4 **(See color insert)** Normal esophageal epithelium and the gastroesophageal junction, which has been opened slightly by gentle insufflation. The gastroesophageal junction is that point where the gastric mucosal folds end to meet the esophageal mucosa.

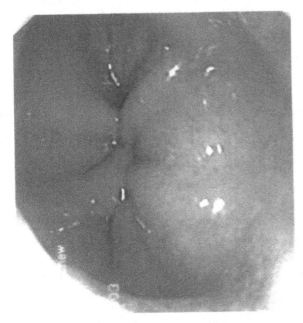

Figure 2.5 **(See color insert)** Hiatal Hernia. Gastric mucosa is above the crural narrowing and there is a ring at the squamocolumnar junction above the crura.

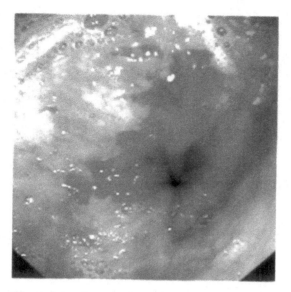

Figure 2.6 (**See color insert**) Suspected short-segment Barrett's esophagus. Gastric epithelium appears above the crural impression and the squamocolumnar junction is irregular. Biopsies are essential to confirm any suspicion for intestinalized epithelium.

1.4. Glycogenic Acanthosis

Small whitish papules are frequently seen in the esophageal mucosa, especially distally. Histologically these are hyperplastic areas of acanthotic epithelium with increased glycogen content. The cause is unknown and has even been ascribed to GERD. The differential diagnosis includes candida infection, leukoplakia, and early cancer.

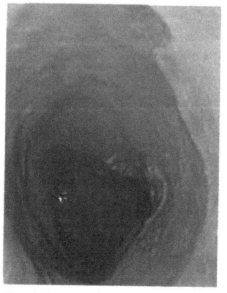

Figure 2.7 (**See color insert**) Long segment Barrett's esophagus confirmed by histological examination.

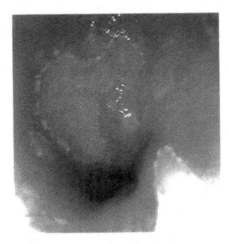

Figure 2.8 **(See color insert)** Barrett's esophagus following a Nissen fundoplication. Squamous islands cover parts of the columnar epithelium in an irregular pattern.

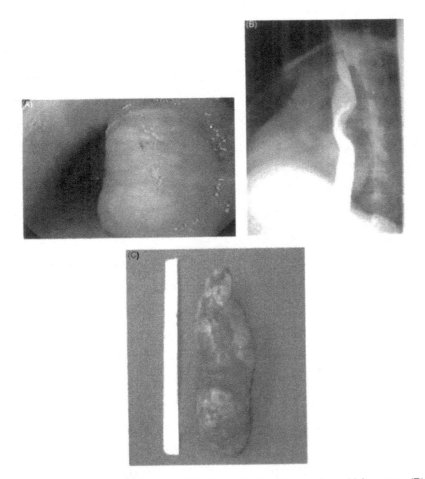

Figure 2.9 **(See color insert)** (A) Endoscopic view of an esophageal leiomyoma. (B) Radiographic appearance of the leiomyoma. (C) The resected specimen.

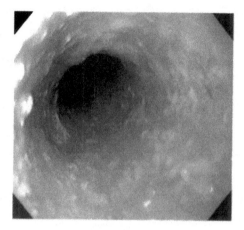

Figure 2.10 **(See color insert)** Monilia infection of the esophagus, which is sometimes seen in achalasia, possibly related to stasis, and in immuno-compromised patients.

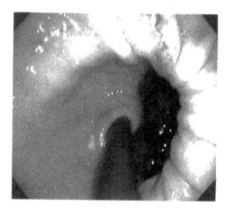

Figure 2.11 **(See color insert)** A large type III hiatal hernia is seen on a retroflexed view of the gastroesophageal junction. The gastroesophageal junction is clearly well above the ring of the hiatus.

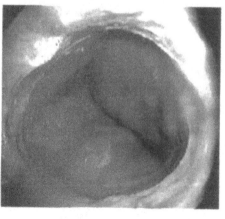

Figure 2.12 **(See color insert)** A small nodule in a short segment Barrett's esophagus proved to be an adenocarcinoma on biopsy.

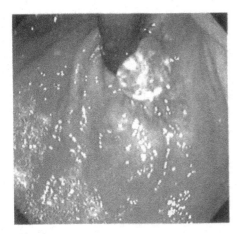

Figure 2.13   **(See color insert)** Retroflexed view of the cardia shows a small nodule, which proved to be an adenocarcinoma on biopsy. This demonstrates the importance of retroflexed viewing of the cardia.

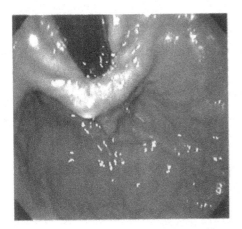

Figure 2.14   **(See color insert)** Retroflexed view of the gastroesophageal junction following a Nissen fundoplication operation. There is a good fit of the 9 mm endoscope on an insufflation. The neovalve does not open up.

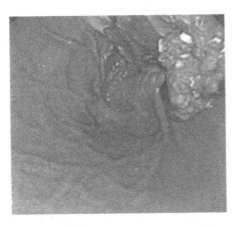

Figure 2.15   **(See color insert)** Post Nissen fundoplication gastric bezoar. A gastric emptying study and tests for vagal integrity are indicated.

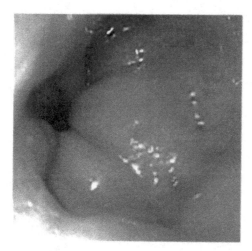

Figure 2.16 **(See color insert)** Endoscopic view of a recurrent hernia following an antireflux operation. Gastric mucosal folds are seen above the hiatus.

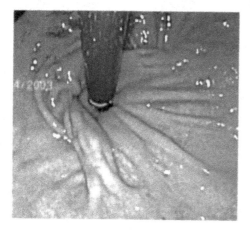

Figure 2.17 **(See color insert)** Retroflexed view of the same patient. The valve is flattened and with insufflation it opens up (Hill's grade III).

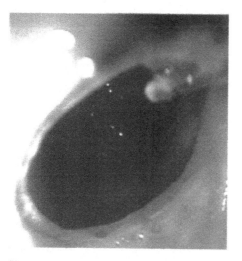

Figure 2.18 **(See color insert)** Healthy mucosa at a cervical esophagogastric anastomosis.

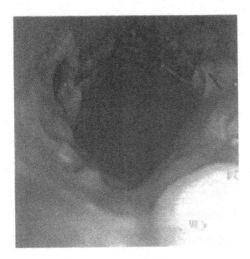

Figure 2.19 (See color insert) Necrotic esophagocolonic anastomosis seen in the early post-operative period. It may be necessary to gently pass a scope as early as the 3rd postoperative day if clinical signs and judgment suggest graft necrosis.

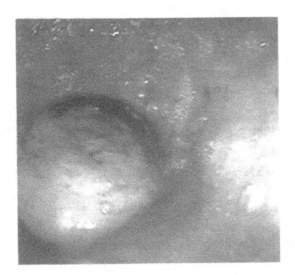

Figure 2.20 (See color insert) Achalasia. There is dilatation of the esophagus and retention of food despite a 2-day "liquid only" diet prior to endoscopy. There may be slight resistance of the lower sphincter, and with careful and slight pressure the endoscope "pops" into the stomach. In early achalasia the esophagus is not dilated and there may not be apparent lower esophageal sphincter resistance. If the patient has dysphagia, and endoscopy appears to be normal, esophageal motility is mandatory to exclude achalasia.

REFERENCES

Boyce HW. Endoscopic definition of esophagogastric junction regional anatomy. Gastrointest Endosc 2000; 51(5): 586–592.

Briel JW, Tamhankar AP, Hagen JA, DeMeester SR, Johansson J, Choustoulakis E, Peters JH, Bremner CG, DeMeester TR. Prevalence and risk factors for ischemia, leak, and stricture of esophageal anastomosis: gastric pull-up versus colon interposition. J Am Coll Surg 2004; 198(4):536–541; discussion 541–542.

Goyal RK, Glancy JJ, Spiro HM. Lower esophageal ring. N Engl J Med 1970; 282:1298–1305, 1355–1362.

Sivak MV. Gastroenterologic Endoscopy. Vol. 1. 2nd ed. Sivak MV Jr. ed. Philadelphia: Saunders, 2000.

Vadva MD, Triadafilopoulos G. Glycogenic acanthosis of the esophagus and gastroesophageal reflux. J Clin Gastroenterol 1993; 17:79–83.

2. ESOPHAGITIS: ENDOSCOPIC GRADING

- Los Angeles Classification

   Grade A: Mucosal breaks confined to the mucosal fold, each not longer than 5 mm;

   Grade B: At least one mucosal break longer than 5 mm, confined to the mucosal fold but not continuous between the folds;

   Grade C: Mucosal breaks that are continuous between the tops of mucosal folds;

   Grade D: Extensive mucosal breaks engaging at least 75% of the esophageal circumference.

- Savary–Miller Classification

   Grade I: Single-fold erosive or exudative lesion, oval or linear;

   Grade II: Two folds with multiple erosions or exudative lesions;

   Grade III: Circumferential erosions;

   Grade IV: Stricture, ulcer, or short esophagus;

   Grade V: Barrett's epithelium.

- Hetzel–Dent Classification

   Grade 0: Normal mucosa;

   Grade I: Mucosal edema, hyperemia, or friability;

   Grade II: Erosions that involve <10% of the lower 5 cm of the esophagus;

   Grade III: Deep ulceration or erosions that involve >50% of the distal esophagus.

- Skinner–Belsey Classification

   Grade I: Mucosal reddening;

   Grade II: Superficial ulceration and membrane formation;

   Grade III: Ulceration, fibrosis, and secondary shortening;

   Grade IV: Mucosa destroyed, fibrosis, shortening, and stricture.

REFERENCES

Armstrong D, Bennet JR, Blum AL et al. The endoscopic assessment of esophagitis: a progress report on observe agreement. Gastroenterology 1996; 111:85–92.

Miller LS. Endoscopy of the esophagus. In: Castell DO, ed. The Esophagus. Boston: Little, Brown & Co., 1995:93–132.

Ollyo JB, Lang F, Fontollet CH et al. Savary's new endoscopic grading of reflux esophagitis: a simple, reproducible, logical, complete, and useful classification. Gastroenterology 1990; 89(suppl A):100.

Skinner DB, Belsey RHR. Surgical management of esophageal reflux and hiatal hernia. J Thorac Cardiovasc Surg 1967; 53(1):33–54.

3
Endoscopic Ultrasonography

Endoscopic ultrasonography (EUS) combines endoscopy and 5–12 MHz frequency ultrasonography to give an evaluation of the different layers of the esophageal wall and adjacent structures outside the wall. The addition of fine needle aspiration (FNA) has enhanced the accuracy of cancer staging. Accurate staging of esophageal cancer is essential to guide therapy. In the study by Clarke et al. (1) positive nodal metastases were present in 33% of intramucosal tumors, 67% of intramural tumors, and 89% of transmural tumors. It is also important to know the status of the celiac nodes before operation, because celiac metastases indicate a very poor prognosis.

The esophagus is also used as a conduit for imaging and biopsy of nodes in the investigation of lung cancer. The sensitivity and specificity for lung cancer diagnosis are 95% and 99% respectively.

1. INSTRUMENTATION

Two systems are available: (1) a radial scanning system which produces a B-mode 360° real-time ultrasound image (7.5–12 MHz) and (2) a 100° curved linear array using 5–7 MHz transducers to provide images parallel to the long axis of the endoscope. This is useful to have a continuous visualization of a needle track used for biopsy of tumors.

The radial scanning system is the usual system used to evaluate the esophageal wall.

The image is perpendicular to the long axis of the endoscope, and the depth of penetration ranges from 6 to 9 mm. A water-filled latex balloon is attached to the ultrasound transducer to allow for acoustic coupling.

Five ultrasonographic layers of the esophageal wall were described by Kimmey et al. (2).

Layer	Echogenicity
Superficial mucosa	Hyper-echoic
Deep mucosa	Hypo-echoic
Submucosa	Hyper-echoic
Muscularis propria	Hypo-echoic
Adventitia	Hyper-echoic

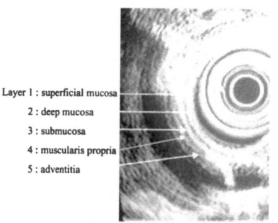

Layer 1 : superficial mucosa
2 : deep mucosa
3 : submucosa
4 : muscularis propria
5 : adventitia

Figure 3.1 Ultrasonographic features of the esophageal wall showing the five layers.

The esophagus is best examined with the balloon technique, when only three of the five layers are often visualized because the balloon effaces the other layers.

2. USES

1. Evaluation of tumor location, extent and depth of wall penetration; Esophageal cancer is a hypo-echoic lesion. EUS gives a better assessment of smaller tumors, whereas CT gives a better assessment of larger tumors;
2. Assessment of periesophageal lymph node metastases which are recognized as being well defined and hypo-echoic;
3. Assessment of mediastinal malignancy;
4. Assessment of pseudo-achalasia;
5. Diagnosis of duplication cyst;
6. Assessment of the extent of benign subepithelial tumors (leiomyoma).

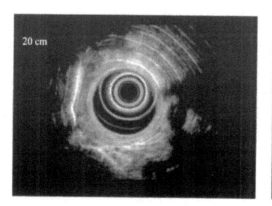
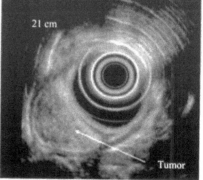

Figure 3.2 Ultrasonographic picture of a tumor of the esophagus at 20 and 21 cm from the incisor teeth. The tumor involves all the layers of the wall. The histology of the resected specimen (esophagectomy) proved this to be a "liposarcoma."

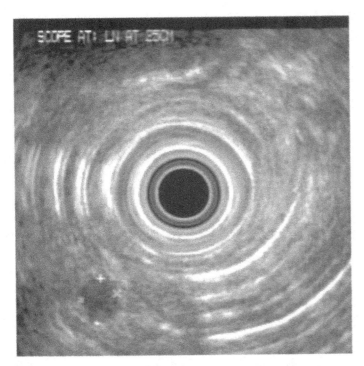

Figure 3.3   Ultrasonographic picture of a lymph node at 25 cm from the incisor teeth in a patient with esophageal carcinoma.

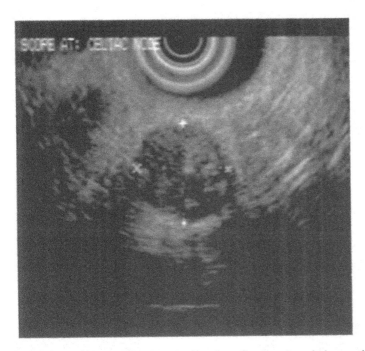

Figure 3.4   Ultrasonographic picture of a celiac lymph node in a patient who had esophageal carcinoma.

2.1. Other Uses

1. EUS has been used to detect muscle thickness in achalasia. A regular thickening of the esophageal wall, water retention, and dilatation of the distal esophagus were noted (3).
2. Eosinophilic esophagitis: Significant expansion of the esophageal wall and individual layers including the combined mucosa, submucosa, and muscularis propria has been demonstrated in children with eosinophilic esophagitis (4).
3. The relationship between esophageal muscle thickness and intraluminal pressure has also been studied. A positive correlation between pressure and muscle thickness was determined (5).

3. CARCINOMA OF THE ESOPHAGUS AND ESOPHAGOGASTRIC JUNCTION

EUS is a valuable method for staging esophageal cancer (6–8). In a study, total accuracy for T-staging of the tumor was about 60%, and accuracy for the detection of transmural growth was about 80% (9). In a larger study, the sensitivity and specificity of EUS detection for esophageal involvement were 89% and 96%, respectively, and for lymph node metastases 85% and 86%, respectively. EUS was not sensitive for detecting extra-esophageal infiltration to mediastinal organs or for the determination of the extent of intra-abdominal spread (10). The accuracy for the detection of nonmetastatic nodes is low (56%).

3.1. Clinical Correlation

Nickl et al. (11) reporting for the American Endosonography Group, showed that EUS changed the treatment plan in 74% of 420 patients evaluated for both benign and malignant diseases.

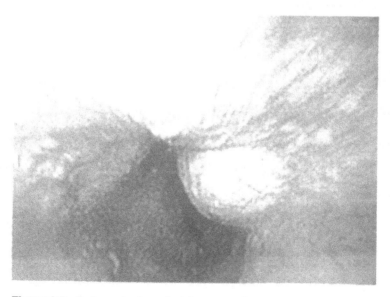

Figure 3.5   Endoscopic view of a leiomyoma of the esophagus. The mucosa is intact.

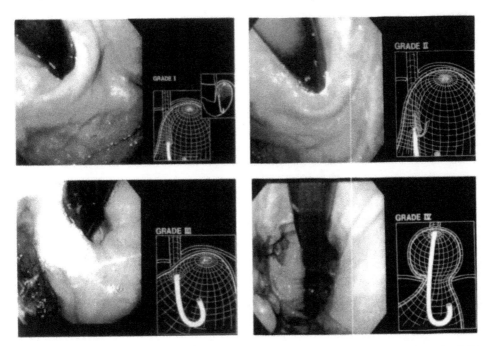

Figure 2.1 Hill's grading of the retroflexed view of the cardia. (With permission from Hill, Lucius D, Kozarek RA. The gastro-esophageal flap valve. J Clin Gastroenterol 1999; 28(3):194–197. *Grade I valve.* A ridge of tissue 3–4 cm long on the lesser curve is closely applied to the endoscope. *Grade II valve.* The ridge is less well defined than in Grade I and it opens occasionally with respiration but closes promptly. *Grade III valve.* The ridge is barely present and there is often failure to close around the endoscope. It is nearly always accompanied by a hiatal hernia and esophagitis. *Grade IV valve.* There is no muscular ridge. The gastroesophageal junction remains open all the time, and the squamous epithelium can often be seen from this retroflexed position. A hiatal hernia is always present.

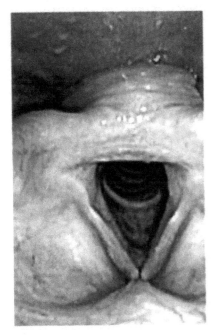

Figure 2.3 View of the normal vocal cords. High gastroesophageal reflux is suspected when posterior redness is seen. The cords are also inspected for movement.

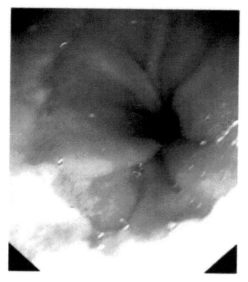

Figure 2.4 Normal esophageal epithelium and the gastroesophageal junction, which has been opened slightly by gentle insufflation. The gastroesophageal junction is that point where the gastric mucosal folds end to meet the esophageal mucosa.

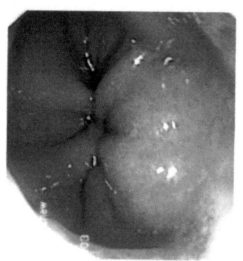

Figure 2.5 Hiatal Hernia. Gastric mucosa is above the crural narrowing and there is a ring at the squamocolumnar junction above the crura.

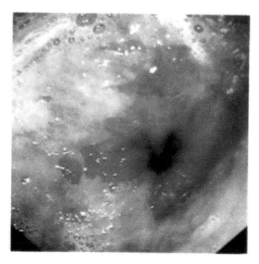

Figure 2.6 Suspected short-segment Barrett's esophagus. Gastric epithelium appears above the crural impression and the squamocolumnar junction is irregular. Biopsies are essential to confirm any suspicion for intestinalized epithelium.

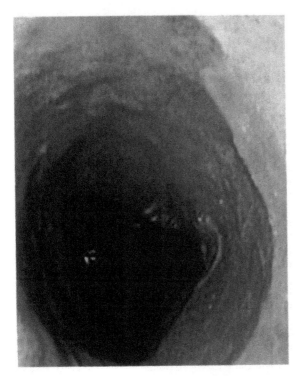

Figure 2.7 Long segment Barrett's esophagus confirmed by histological examination.

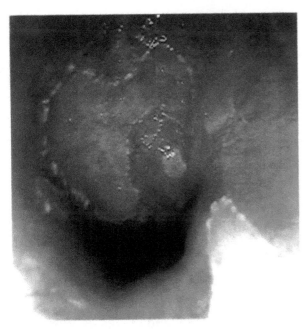

Figure 2.8 Barrett's esophagus following a Nissen fundoplication. Squamous islands cover parts of the columnar epithelium in an irregular pattern.

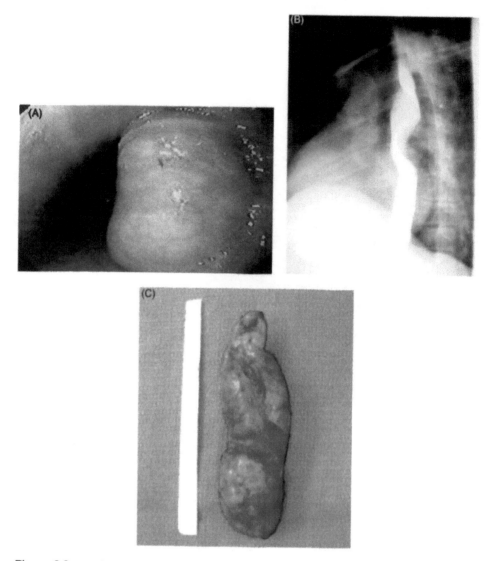

Figure 2.9 (A) Endoscopic view of an esophageal leiomyoma. (B) Radiographic appearance of the leiomyoma. (C) The resected specimen.

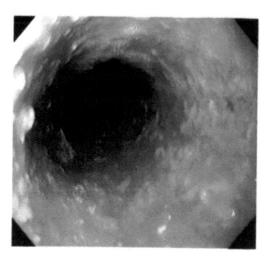

Figure 2.10 Monilia infection of the esophagus, which is sometimes seen in achalasia, possibly related to stasis, and in immuno-compromised patients.

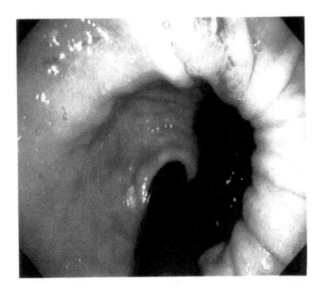

Figure 2.11 A large type III hiatal hernia is seen on a retroflexed view of the gastroesophageal junction. The gastroesophageal junction is clearly well above the ring of the hiatus.

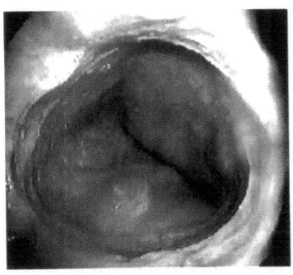

Figure 2.12 A small nodule in a short segment Barrett's esophagus proved to be an adenocarcinoma on biopsy.

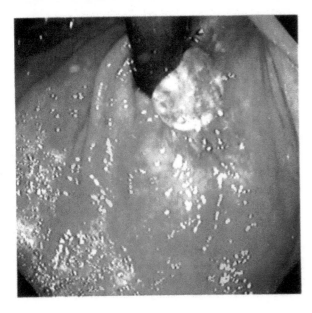

Figure 2.13 Retroflexed view of the cardia shows a small nodule, which proved to be an adenocarcinoma on biopsy. This demonstrates the importance of retroflexed viewing of the cardia.

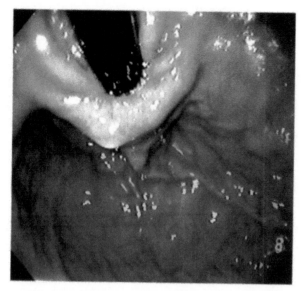

Figure 2.14 Retroflexed view of the gastroesophageal junction following a Nissen fundoplication operation. There is a good fit of the 9 mm endoscope on an insufflation. The neovalve does not open up.

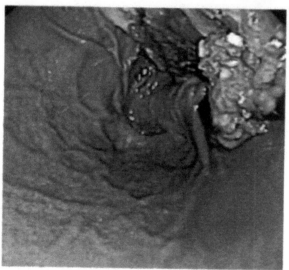

Figure 2.15 Post Nissen fundoplication gastric bezoar. A gastric emptying study and tests for vagal integrity are indicated.

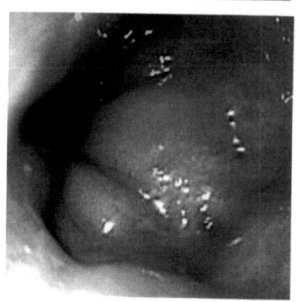

Figure 2.16 Endoscopic view of a recurrent hernia following an antireflux operation. Gastric mucosal folds are seen above the hiatus.

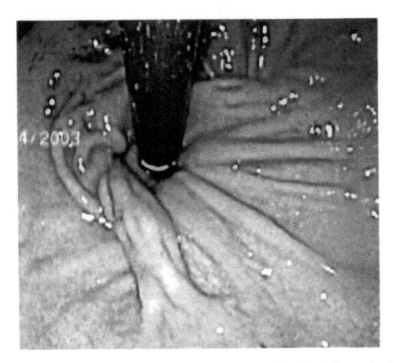

Figure 2.17 Retroflexed view of the same patient. The valve is flattened and with insufflation it opens up (Hill's grade III).

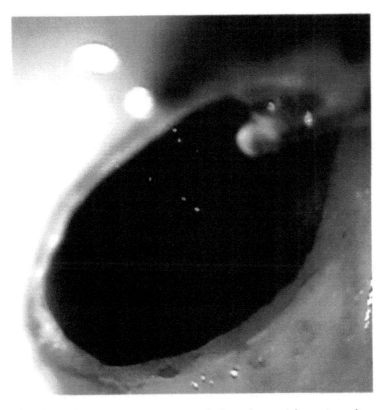

Figure 2.18 Healthy mucosa at a cervical esophagogastric anastomosis.

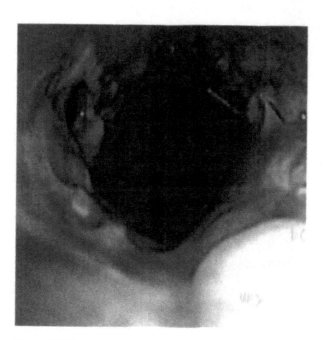

Figure 2.19 Necrotic esophagocolonic anastomosis seen in the early postoperative period. It may be necessary to gently pass a scope as early as the 3rd postoperative day if clinical signs and judgment suggest graft necrosis.

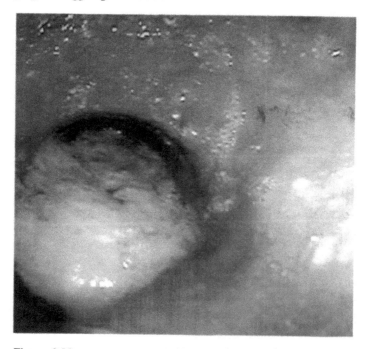

Figure 2.20 Achalasia. There is dilatation of the esophagus and retention of food despite a 2-day "liquid only" diet prior to endoscopy. There may be slight resistance of the lower sphincter, and with careful and slight pressure the endoscope "pops" into the stomach. In early achalasia the esophagus is not dilated and there may not be apparent lower esophageal sphincter resistance. If the patient has dysphagia, and endoscopy appears to be normal, esophageal motility is mandatory to exclude achalasia.

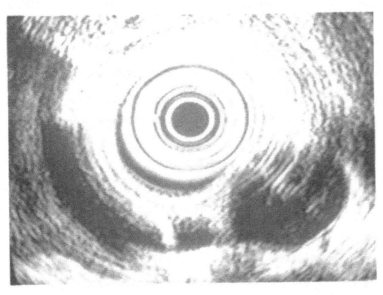

Figure 3.6 Endoscopic ultrasound appearances of the leiomyoma. The mucosal layer is compressed but is not infiltrated.

On the basis of preoperative EUS patients were selected for curative or palliative resection of esophageal cancer. The results of a study at University of Southern California (12) were as follows:

Tumor length: correct prediction 85%
Wall penetration: accurate prediction 76%
Regional lymph nodes: accurate prediction 82%

Using the WNM [wall penetration (W), lymph nodes (N), systemic metastases (M)] staging system, EUS correctly staged the cancer in 68% of patients.

Wallace et al. (13) analyzed multiple staging management strategies for carcinoma of the esophagus, including CT, EUS, PET, and thorascopy/laparoscopy, and concluded that PET scanning plus EUS with FNA was the recommended staging procedure for patients with esophageal carcinoma. If PET is unavailable, CT plus EUS with FNA is preferred.

REFERENCES

1. Clarke GWB, Peters JH, Ireland AP, Ehsan A, Hagen JA, Kiyabu MT, Bremner CG, DeMeester TR. Nodal metastases and sites of recurrence after en bloc esophagectomy for adenocarcinoma. Ann Thorac Surg 1994; 58:646–654.
2. Kimmey MB, Martin RW, Haggi RC et al. Histologic correlates of gastrointestinal ultrasound images. Gastroenterology 1989; 96:433–441.
3. Sezkin O, Ulker A, Temucin G. Sonographic findings in achalasia. J Clin Ultrasound 2001; 1:31–40.
4. Fox VL, Nurko S, Teitelbaum JE, Badizadegan K, Furuta GT. High resolution EUS in children with eosinophilic "allergic" esophagitis. Gastrointest Endosc 2003; 57:30–36.
5. Pehlivanov N, Liu J, Kassab GS, Puckett JL, Ittal R. Relationship between esophageal muscle thickness and intraluminal pressure: an ultrasonographic study. AJP—Gastrointest Liver Phys 2001; 280:G1093–G1098.

6. Botet JF, Lightdale CJ. Endoscopic sonography of the upper gastrointestinal tract. Am J Roentgenol 1991; 156:63–68.
7. Nikl NJ, Cotton PD. Clinical application of endoscopic ultrasonography. Am J Gastroenterol 1990; 85:675–682.
8. Lightdale CJ. Staging of esophageal cancer. 1. Endoscopic ultrasonography. Semin Oncol 1994; 21:438–446.
9. Hiele M, Leyn P, Schurmans P, Lerut A, Huys S, Geboes K, Gevers AM, Rutgeets P. Relation between endoscopic ultrasound findings and outcome of patients with tumors of the esophagus or esophagogastric junction. Gastrointest Endosc 1997; 45:381–386.
10. Fok M, Cheng SW, Wong J. Endosonography in patient selection for surgical treatment of esophageal carcinoma. World J Surg 1992; 16:1098–1103.
11. Nickl NJ, Bhutani MS, Catalano M et al. Clinical implications of endoscopic ultrasonography: the American Endosonography Study. Gastrointest Endosc 1996; 44(4):371–377.
12. Peters JH, Hoeft SF, Heimbucher J, Bremner RM, DeMeester TR, Bremner CG, Clark GWB, Kiyabu M, Parisky Y. Selection of patients for curative or palliative resection based on preoperative endoscopic ultrasonography. Arch Surg 1994; 129:534–539.
13. Wallace MB, Nietert PJ, Earle C, Krasna MJ, Hawes RH, Hoffman BJ, Reed CE. An analysis of multiple staging management strategies for carcinoma of the esophagus: computed tomography, endoscopic ultrasonography, positron emission tomography and thorascopy/laparoscopy. Ann Thorac Surg 2002; 74:1026–1032.

4

Esophageal Manometry

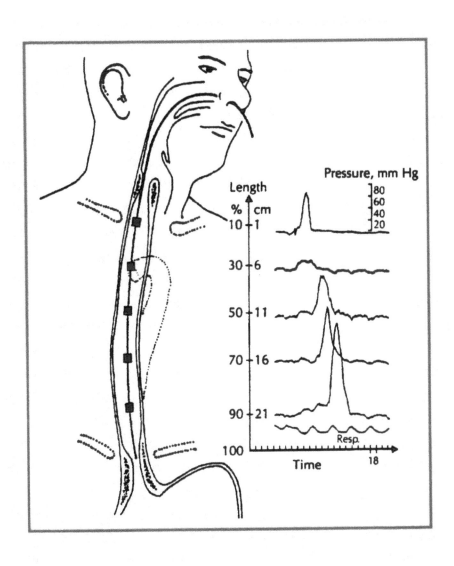

1. INDICATIONS FOR ESOPHAGEAL MANOMETRY

- *Diagnostic*
  Motility disorders: achalasia, scleroderma, nutcracker esophagus, diffuse esophageal spasm (DES), hypertensive lower esophageal sphincter (HLES), ineffective esophageal motility (IEM), nonspecific esophageal motor disorder (NSEMD).
  Dysphagia: assessment of the cause of functional obstruction.
  Chest pain: assessment of the cause and relation to gastroesophageal reflux.
  Respiratory disorders: assessment of abnormal motility associated with gastroesophageal reflux.
- *Preoperative assessment*
  Verification of the correct diagnosis and suitability for surgery.
  Avoidance of postoperative dysphagia.
- *Postoperative assessment*
  Assessment of the response to surgery.
  Assessment of the cause of failed surgery.
- *Investigational*

2. ESOPHAGEAL FUNCTION LABORATORY

Location. The laboratory can be located in the clinic or hospital. The endoscopy suite is an ideal location and the same technicians or nurses can assist with both procedures. The room requires a basin and water supply. Cleaning apparatus is best installed in an adjacent room.

Personnel. A trained technician or nurse can perform the procedure. Supervision by a doctor is advisable for difficult cases or difficult intubations such as that may occur with achalasia.

Equipment. Reliable and excellent manufacturers supply modern state-of-the-art equipment. After-service is crucial to the smooth running and updating of the programs. Medtronic Inc. and Sandhill Scientific Inc. are the leaders in the USA.

3. MOTILITY LABORATORY EQUIPMENT

1. Multichannel motility system (Polygraf 1.0) with respiration and swallow sensors (Medtronic Gastroenterology, Minn.).
2. Hydraulic capillary infusion system with an infusion rate of 0.5 cc/min (Arndorfer Medical Specialties, Greendale, WI) (Mui Scientific).
3. Water-perfused multilumen manometric catheter with 0.8 mm lateral openings placed 5 cm apart and radially orientated 72 from each other and 75 cm long (Arndorfer Medical Specialties, Greendale, WI) (Mui Scientific) can be built to meet the specific requirements.
4. Solid-state manometric catheter can be built to meet the requirements (Konigsburg Instruments). This is optional.

5. Puller apparatus for slow motorized pull-through (sMPT) assessment of LES (Medtronic, Inc).
6. Solid-state catheters: these are more expensive and less robust. They are used for ambulatory motility.

Water-perfused systems require a capillary water perfusion apparatus (Arndorfer). Water-perfused catheters are much cheaper than solid-state catheters. Solid-state catheters are expensive but do not require a water-perfusion system. The Dent sleeve catheter assembly simplifies the evaluation of relaxation of the LES, but has the disadvantage that sphincter length cannot be assessed. pH testing requires special ambulatory apparatus. Disposable probes or reusable glass probes are options. Glass probes have less asterixis and are more reliable in detection of alkaline pH. Both are reliable for the detection of acid exposure. A catheter-free pH monitoring system (Bravo) is now available and a description is included in the chapter on pH monitoring.

4. PATIENT PREPARATION AND PASSAGE OF THE MANOMETRY CATHETER*

4.1. Patient Preparation

Preparation of the patient is essential in order to obtain a useful manometric study. In the clinic, or during a telephone interview, the patient's knowledge level of the contemplated procedure should be assessed. If the patient is being referred from an outside clinic, an explanation as to what the test involves may not be given. A thorough explanation of what the procedure involves and the discomfort level the patient can expect allows the patient to begin a mental preparation for the study. Questions can also be answered at this time and misconceptions regarding the procedure can be corrected. Decreasing anxiety levels before and during the procedure greatly enhance the results of the study.

The patient should be instructed to be NPO at least 6 h before the study. Prokinetic agents and calcium channel blockers should be discontinued 72 h before the manometric study. If a 24 h pH study is being performed after the manometry, we recommend that proton pump inhibitors be discontinued for 14 days before the test, H2 blockers 72 h and antacids 24 h prior to the test.

In our laboratory we find it helpful if the patient has had a recent videoesophagram, upper gastrointestinal series, or upper gastrointestinal endoscopy before the manometry. If the presence of a stricture, diverticulum, large hiatal hernia or paraesophageal hernia, or dilated or bird-beak esophagus is known before an attempt is made to pass the manometry catheter it can sometimes explain problems encountered along the way.

4.2. Manometry Catheter Insertion

Patient NPO status and whether the patient discontinued the requested medications have to be ascertained. Informed consent and a brief patient history should be obtained. The patient has to be inquired as to whether the patient has ever had any nasal trauma or

---

*Sue Corkill (Foregut function laboratory director, USC Department of Surgery).

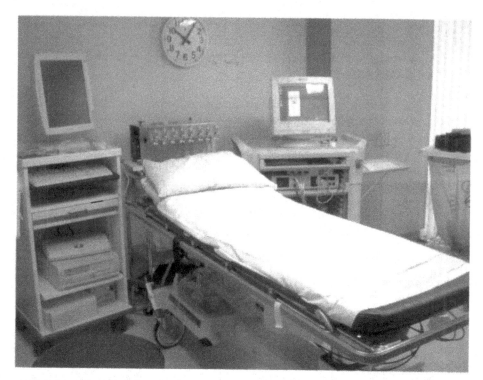

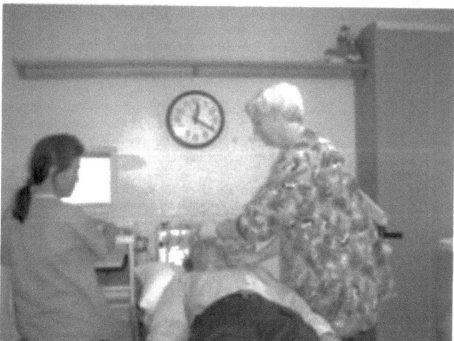

Figure 4.1 (Upper) The esophageal manometry laboratory. A perfusion pump is used for water-perfused catheters. The apparatus for the motorized pull-through is seen in the background. (Lower) Esophageal manometry in progress. A stationary pull-through (SPT) study is being performed, and the manometry catheter is pulled from the stomach in 1 cm increments. The recordings are visualized on the computer screen and saved for computerized evaluation.

nasal surgeries. The patient should be explained how the catheter is going to be inserted and what they can expect to feel during the insertion. Patients have to be reassured that they will be able to breathe and that some gagging is normal and should be expected, but will get better. They should also be explained that they will feel the pressure when the catheter is inserted in the nose and that they will feel the presence of the catheter in the back of the throat.

Both nares are anesthetized with 2% topical xylocaine jelly or 4% topical cocaine solution, depending on the physician's preference. After allowing sufficient time for the anesthetic to work, the patient is made to sit up for the tube insertion. A towel is placed in the patients lap, and an emesis basin, tissues, and water should be kept ready. The patient is asked to tilt the chin up slightly, and the lubricated catheter is gently advanced into the selected nostril. The catheter is advanced straight back, not upwards, until it passes into the hypopharynx. A decrease in resistance can usually be felt at this point, and the patient may also gag. The patient is asked to gently tilt the chin down onto the chest, and instructed to hold a glass of water to and take sips of water using the straw. As the patient swallows, the catheter is advanced through the cricopharyngeus muscle area (crico). One should be able to feel the catheter pass through the crico and into the esophagus. If the patient begins coughing uncontrollably and is unable to talk, the trachea might have been intubated. The catheter is withdrawn gently until it is in the hypopharynx, the patient's head is repositioned with the chin down on the chest and the catheter is passed again. After it reaches the esophagus, the patient is asked to stop drinking and take some deep breaths to relax. If the patient is gagging uncontrollably, a flashlight and tongue blade are used to check the back of the throat to see if the catheter is curling in the mouth. If this occurs, the catheter is gently withdrawn into the hypopharynx and begun again. Once the tip of the catheter is past the back of the throat, gagging will lessen. After a moment, the catheter is gently advanced and if drinking water seems to help, the patient is instructed to continue to swallow the water. When the catheter has passed through the hiatus into the distal esophagus, slow, gentle, steady pressure will usually allow the catheter to pass through into the stomach. Once the end-point of the catheter is reached and the catheter is in the stomach, it is gently taped to the patient's nose.

The easiest way to verify the position of the catheter is to connect it to the transducers (if a water-perfused system is used) or connect the solid-state catheter to the recording device and turn the system on. If all sensors are in the stomach, a gastric baseline pressure with positive, shallow deflections upon inspiration is observed. If the catheter is coiled in the esophagus, negative deflections upon inspiration and esophageal contractions is observed when the patient swallows. If the catheter is coiled in the esophagus, the catheter is gently pulled back until it unkinks and then passed again. Generally the catheter does not have to be removed completely. Complications of catheter insertion include epistaxis, tracheal intubation, aspiration, and esophageal or gastric perforation.

4.3. Special Situations

4.3.1. Achalasia

A prior videoesophagram is essential. If the esophagus is large, dilated, and/or tortuous, it will be almost impossible to pass the manometry catheter without endoscopic guidance. If the esophagus is mildly dilated, the catheter can usually be passed without endoscopic help. These patients should be approached on an individual basis. For patients with suspected achalasia, chill the catheter by placing it in a plastic bag in the freezer compartment of a refrigerator or use a "stiffer" catheter. These stiffer catheters will sometimes pass more easily through a dilated esophagus or a HLES. Patience is the keyword and if one sensor is passed through the lower esophageal sphincter (LES), it is easy to get the rest through.

After initial intubation (i.e., through the cricopharyngeus), the patient is asked to lie down and the catheter is connected to the recording device so as to detect exactly where the catheter is. Sometimes having the patient lie on the left and/or right sides will facilitate the passage of the catheter. If some of the sensors are through the LES (as evidenced by a gastric baseline pressure) and the end of the catheter has been reached, the catheter is gently withdrawn to uncoil it, being careful not to pull the most proximal sensor that is in the stomach back out into the esophagus, and then gently advance the catheter again. Repeat this as many times as needed until all sensors are in the stomach.

4.3.2. Hiatal Hernia

Patients with hiatal hernia can also present a challenge to the passage of the manometry catheter. Hernias <5 cm can usually be navigated without any difficulty. With larger hernias, the catheter has a tendency to coil in the hernia and not pass below the diaphragm. Endoscopic placement may be necessary for these patients with very large hernias. Again, each patient should be approached on an individual basis, and if difficulty is encountered while trying to pass the catheter through the larger hernias, the patient is asked to stand up or lie on either side to facilitate the passage.

4.3.3. Paraesophageal Hernia/Intrathoracic Stomach

The same problems encountered with a large hiatal hernia can also be present for those patients with a paraesophageal hernia or those with an intrathoracic stomach. In most patients the catheter can be passed without endoscopic guidance. If it is observed that the catheter passes without difficulty into the stomach, then the gastric baseline may show a negative pressure because part or all of the stomach may be exposed to the negative pressure of the chest. There should be no esophageal contractions when the patient swallows, or an X-ray is obtained to verify the catheter position.

4.3.4. Zenker Diverticulum

A videoesophagram before manometry is essential for anyone with a suspected Zenker diverticulum. It is virtually impossible to pass the catheter without endoscopic guidance on someone who has a large Zenker's. It is usually possible to navigate past a smaller diverticulum. Again, each patient should be approached on an individual basis. When passing the motility catheter, resistance usually indicates that the catheter is coiling in the diverticulum. Gently withdraw the catheter until it is in the hypopharynx and try again. It is sometimes better to not have the patient drink water while trying to pass the catheter. Fiberoptic endoscopic guidance may be necessary to pass a guide-wire or catheter into the esophageal opening in order to place the manometry catheter.

4.3.5. Epiphrenic and Mid-Esophageal Diverticulum

Patients with these types of diverticula will generally require endoscopic placement of the catheter. Again, size and location of the diverticulum will determine whether to place the catheter endoscopically or not.

4.3.6. Passage and Position of Catheters for Ambulatory and pH Studies

For placement of ambulatory catheters we recommend performing stationary esophageal manometry first in order to define the manometric location of the LES and then to position the catheter. For esophageal pH and ambulatory manometry, the catheter should be positioned 5 cm above the upper border of the LES. Fluoroscopy, endoscopy, and/or pH change placement methods are not accurate and should not be used. Height formulas are appropriate for children but not for adults.

These catheters are passed in the same fashion as the manometry catheter. As these catheters are generally smaller in diameter than the manometry catheter, they curl more easily. We recommend passing all pH catheters down into the stomach initially (verified by the pH) and then pulling the catheter back to the predetermined position. This will ensure that the catheter is not curled in the esophagus. An X-ray can also confirm the position.

Table 4.1 Manometric Features of Primary Esophageal Motility Disorders

LES		Esophageal body	
Achalasia			
Baseline pressure	Relaxation	Baseline	Peristalsis
Elevated (>27 mmHg) may be normal in ~50% patients	Incomplete (residual pressure >7.5 mmHg)	Elevated	Absent
DES			
May be abnormal		>20% simultaneous contractions—main feature	
Nutcracker Esophagus			
Normal, hypertensive, or nonrelaxing		Mean pressures of swallow responses >180 mmHg Responses may be of a long duration (mean >6 s) Normal peristaltic progression	
Hypertensive LES			
Resting pressure elevated (>27 mmHg)	Relaxation may be normal or incomplete	Normal peristaltic progression "Ramp"intrabolus pressure may be raised in distal esophagus.	
"Scleroderma" (progressive systemic sclerosis)			
Resting pressures are low Poor swallow responses normal coordination		Hypomotile Normal cricopharyngeal sphincter [low crico pressures in polymyositis and mixed connective tissue disease (MCTD)].	

(continued)

Table 4.1 *Continued*

LES	Esophageal body
Nonspecific esophageal motility disorders (NEMD) *(any combination of abnormalities below)*	
Incomplete relaxation (<90%) or (residual pressure 7.5 mmHg)	Nontransmitted contractions (>20%) Triple peaked contractions Retrograde contractions Low amplitude (mean <35 mmHg) Prolonged duration (mean >6 s)
IEM Normal or low pressure	>30% responses have <30 mmHg pressure >30% responses are nontransmitted

5. CLASSIFICATION OF ESOPHAGEAL MANOMETRIC ABNORMALITIES AFTER SPECHLER AND CASTELL*

- Inadequate LES relaxation
  - Classical achalasia
  - Atypical disorders of LES relaxation
- Uncoordinated contraction
  - Diffuse esophageal spasm
- Hypercontraction
  - Nutcracker esophagus
  - Isolated hypertensive LES
- Hypocontraction
  - Ineffective esophageal motility

6. BARRIER TO REFLUX: THE PHYSIOLOGICAL BASIS FOR SURGICAL ANTIREFLUX THERAPY

6.1. History of Surgical Antireflux Therapy

Antireflux surgery is a relatively modern form of therapy for gastroesophageal reflux disease (GERD). It was initiated in the 1950s when Dr. Allison (1) recognized an association between a hiatal hernia and reflux esophagitis. He focused attention on the repair of the hernia, but the long-term outcome was of minimal benefit. Antireflux surgery assumed a more physiological therapeutic role in the late 1970s when it was shown that a complete or partial fundoplication could correct a defective LES, heal

*Spechler SJ, Castell DO. Classification of oesophageal motility abnormalities. Gut 2001; 49(1): 145–151.

advanced mucosal injury, and control disease difficult to manage by medical therapy. During the 1980s the outcome of antireflux procedures was improved by defining the indication for surgical therapy and standardizing the surgical technique. The advances in minimally invasive surgery in the 1990s allowed antireflux procedures to be performed laparoscopically. The Nissen fundoplication became the most common antireflux procedure done laparoscopically with more than 70,000 performed annually. More than 5000 patient outcomes following laparoscopic Nissen fundoplication have been reported with a success rate of 94%, a postoperative morbidity rate of 2%, and a mortality of less than 0.1% (2). The laparoscopic approach provided definitive treatment, improved patient comfort, shorter hospital stay, less convalescence, and a more acceptable cosmetic result. Today, endoscopic antireflux procedures are just beginning to be introduced. What role they play in the treatment of early or advanced GERD is yet to be determined. At present, the laparoscopic Nissen fundoplication is particularly effective in patients with early reflux disease and has become the "gold standard" to which the results of endoscopic procedures must be compared.

The principle pathophysiological abnormality responsible for symptomatic gastroesophageal reflux is the failure of the barrier or valve between the stomach and esophagus. Under normal conditions there is a pressure gradient between the abdomen and the thorax: the pressure in the abdomen is higher in the abdomen than in the thorax (Fig. 4.2). If the barrier or valve is absent, free flow of gastric juice from the stomach into the esophagus can occur unabated. Surgical repair of a failed barrier, whether through an open incision or a laparoscope, corrects the cause of GERD and has the ability to alter the natural history of the disease. In contrast, acid suppression therapy alters the pH of the gastric juice refluxed through the defective barrier in an effort to control the symptoms of the

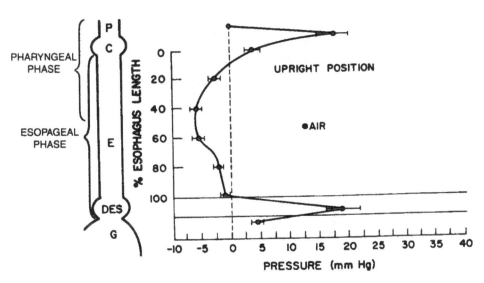

Figure 4.2 Diagrammatic representation of the esophageal pressure profile in the upright position, detected by a water-perfused catheter withdrawal from the stomach and through the esophagus and sphincters. Intragastric pressure is about 5 mmHg and the peak pressure in the LES is below 20 mmHg. The intrathoracic pressure is negative to intragastric pressure and the negativity is greatest in the mid-esophagus. The pressure becomes positive again in the upper esophageal sphincter (UES).

disease, but is ineffective at correcting the cause of the disease. If the proposed endoscopic procedures are shown to be effective, even if to a lesser degree than the laparoscopic Nissen fundoplication, they would provide the least invasive approach to correct the cause of reflux and prevent its complications. This has the possibility of shifting the focus of therapy from management to curative.

6.2. Physiology of the Gastroesophageal Barrier

In humans, the barrier that confines the gastric environment to the stomach is the LES. It has no anatomical landmarks, but its presence can be identified by a rise in pressure over gastric baseline pressure when a pressure transducer is pulled from the stomach into the esophagus (Fig. 4.3). This high-pressure zone (HPZ) is normally present except in two situations: after a swallow, when it is momentarily dissipated or relaxes to allow passage of food into the stomach, and during a belch, when it allows gas to be vented from a distended fundus. The common denominator for virtually all episodes of gastroe-sophageal reflux is the loss of the normal HPZ or barrier. When the barrier is absent, resistance to the flow of gastric juice from an environment of higher pressure—the stomach—to an environment of lower pressure—the esophagus—is lost. In early disease, this is usually due to a transient loss of the barrier. In advanced disease, this is usually due to the permanent loss of the barrier (3).

There are three characteristics of this HPZ, commonly referred to as the LES, which maintain its function as a barrier to intragastric and intra-abdominal pressure challenges (Fig. 4.3). Two of these characteristics—the overall length of the sphincter and the sphinc-ter pressure—work together and depend on each other to provide resistance to the flow of gastric juice from the stomach into the esophagus (4). The shorter the overall length, the higher the pressure must be for the sphincter to maintain sufficient resistance to remain competent (4) (Fig. 4.4). Consequently, the effect of a normal sphincter pressure can be nullified by a short overall sphincter length, and the effect of a normal overall sphincter length can be nullified by a low sphincter pressure.

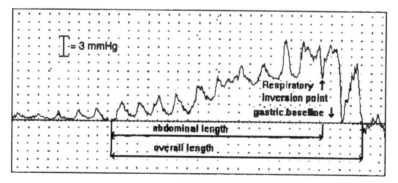

Figure 4.3 A pressure profile of the lower esophageal HPZ or sphincter measured in a normal subject. The HPZ has no anatomical landmarks, but is identified by a rise in pressure over the gastric baseline as a pressure transducer is pulled from the stomach into the esophagus. Note the long intra-abdominal portion identified by the positive respiratory excursions and the short intra-thoracic portion identified by the negative respiratory excursions. The point where the respiratory excursions reverse is called the RIP. Pressure scale is 3 mmHg between vertical dots.

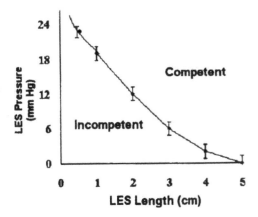

Figure 4.4 The relationship of the sphincter pressure (measured at the RIP) and overall sphincter length to the resistance to the flow of fluid through the barrier. LES, lower esophageal sphincter; competent, no flow; incompetent, flow of varied volumes. Note that the shorter the overall length of the HPZ, the higher the pressures must be to maintain sufficient resistance to remain competent.

For practical purposes, the pressure of the sphincter is measured at a single point—the respiratory inversion point (RIP)—but in actuality, pressure is applied over the entire length of the sphincter. A more accurate assessment of barrier resistance is to measure the radial pressure exerted in four quadrants over the entire length of the sphincter. This allows the computer formation of a three-dimensional image of the sphincter or barrier (Fig. 4.5). The volume of this image reflects the sphincter's resistance to the flow of fluid through it. This is called the "sphincter pressure vector volume" (SPVV). A calculated volume less than the fifth percentile of normal resting subjects is an indication of a permanently defective sphincter (5).

A fundamental principle is that the length of the barrier or sphincter is critical to its function. Shortening of sphincter length occurs naturally with gastric filling, as the terminal esophagus is "taken up" by the expanding fundus (6) (Fig. 4.6). This is similar to the shortening of the neck of a balloon as it is inflated. With excessive gastric distention, the length of the sphincter shortens to a critical point at which it gives way and the pressure drops precipitously and reflux occurs (7) (Fig. 4.7). If the length of the sphincter is permanently short, then further shortening caused by the normal gastric distention with meals will result in postprandial reflux.

The observation that gastric distention results in shortening of the sphincter down to a critical length, so that the pressure dissipates, the lumen opens and reflux occurs, provides a mechanical explanation for "transient sphincter relaxation" without invoking a neuromuscular reflex. If only the sphincter pressure and not its length is measured, as with a Dent sleeve, the event will appear as a spontaneous relaxation of sphincter pressure (8). In reality, it is the progressive shortening of the sphincter, rather than transient relaxations, that results in the loss of sphincter pressure.

Variations in the anatomy of the cardia, from a normal acute angle of His to an abnormal dome architecture of a sliding hiatal hernia, influences the ease with which the sphincter is shortened by gastric distention. Hernia can result from the pulsion force of abdominal pressure on the esophageal hiatus or from the traction produced by inflammatory fibrosis of the esophageal body. The resulting alteration in the geometry

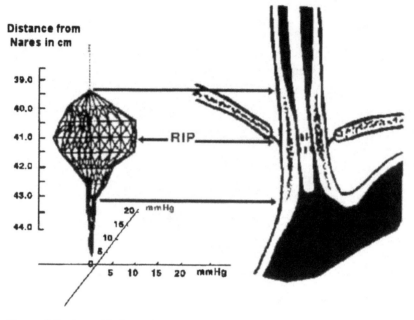

Figure 4.5 A graphic illustration of how a three-dimensional computerized image of the sphincter can be constructed by measuring the pressure of the HPZ in four quadrants at 0.5 cm intervals over the entire length of the zone. The volume of the image reflects the resistance of the sphincter to the flow of gastric juice into the esophagus, and is called the SPVV. [With permission from Stein et al. (5).]

of the cardia places the sphincter at a mechanical disadvantage in maintaining its length with progressive degrees of gastric distention. Greater gastric distention is necessary to open the barrier in patients with an intact angle of His than in those with a hiatal hernia (9). This is because the dome or funnel shape of a hiatal hernia allows the wall tension

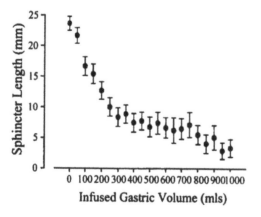

Figure 4.6 The relationship between overall sphincter length and gastric distention with increasing volumes of water. As the gastric volume increases, the sphincter length shortens with the distal esophagus being taken up by the expanding fundus (4).

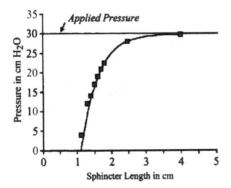

Figure 4.7 The relationship between resting sphincter pressure measured by manometry and sphincter length when applied pressure or "sphincter squeeze" is kept constant. Analysis was made with a model of the lower esophageal HPZ. Note that as sphincter length decreases, the pressure recorded within the sphincter decreases only slightly, until a length of 2 cm is reached, when sphincter pressure drops precipitously and competency of the sphincter is lost. [With permission from Pettersson et al. (7).]

forces that pull open the barrier with gastric distention to be more effectively applied to the gastroesophageal junction (10). This accounts for the common association of a hiatal hernia with GERD. Kahrilas et al. (11) demonstrated this mechanical disadvantage by studying the effect of intragastric air infusion on the number of transient sphincter relaxations or "shortening" per hour. Patients with hiatal hernia had significantly more per hour than control subjects and those without hernias. Intragastric distention with air infusion resulted in a gradual shortening of the sphincter in all three groups. The shortening occurred in a distal to cephalad direction and preceded the loss of sphincter pressure.

The third characteristic of the lower esophageal HPZ or "sphincter" is its position. A portion of the overall length of the HPZ, normally exposed to positive intra-abdominal pressure environment, is commonly referred to as the abdominal length of the sphincter (Fig. 4.2) (12). During the periods of increased intra-abdominal pressure, the resistance of the sphincter would easily be overcome if the position of the sphincter were such that the abdominal pressure was unable to be applied equally to the sphincter and stomach (13–15). Think of sucking on a soft soda straw immersed in a bottle of coke; the positive hydrostatic pressure of the fluid and the negative pressure inside the straw due to sucking cause the straw to collapse instead of allowing the liquid to flow up the straw in the direction of the negative pressure. If the sphincter is positioned so that the abdominal length is inadequate, the sphincter cannot collapse in response to applied positive intra-abdominal pressure and the negative intrathoracic pressure will encourage reflux to occur. Greater than 1 cm of sphincter should be exposed to the abdominal pressure environment in order for it to respond effectively to changes in intra-abdominal pressure (16).

If a sphincter, in the fasting state, has an abnormally low pressure, a short overall length or minimal length exposure to the abdominal pressure environment, the result is a permanent loss of resistance with unhampered reflux of gastric contents into the esophagus. This is known as a permanently defective barrier or sphincter and is identified by one or more of the following characteristics: an average pressure of <6 mmHg, an average overall length of 2 cm or less, and an average length exposed to the positive pressure environment of the abdomen of 1 cm or shorter. Compared with normal subjects, these values are below the 2.5 percentile for each parameter (17). The most common consequence of a permanently defective sphincter is increased esophageal exposure to gastric juice, resulting in inflammatory injury to the mucosa and muscularis propria, causing reduced contraction amplitude and abnormal waveforms in the esophageal body. If the reflux is not brought under control, the progressive loss of effective esophageal clearance results in an ever-increasing esophageal acid exposure (Fig. 4.6) (18–20).

6.3. Causes and Consequences of the Failure of the Gastroesophageal Barrier

Early GERD is initiated by increased transient losses of the barrier secondary to gastric overdistention from excessive air and food ingestion (21,22). The vectors produced by gastric wall tension pull on the gastroesophageal junction, resulting in the terminal esophagus being taken up into the stretched fundus, thereby reducing the length of the sphincter. With overeating, a critical length is reached, usually about 1–2 cm; when the sphincter gives way, its pressure drops precipitously and reflux occurs (Fig. 4.7). If the swallowed air is vented, the length of the sphincter is restored and competency returns until subsequent distention again shortens it and further reflux occurs. Aerophagia is common in patients with GERD because they swallow more frequently in order to use their saliva to neutralize the acid gastric juice refluxed into their esophagus (23). The ingested air results in gastric distention. Together, the actions of overeating and swallowing air result in the common complaint of postprandial bloating, repetitive belching, and heartburn in patients with early GERD. The high prevalence of the disease in the western world is thought to be secondary to the eating habits of western society (24). Gastric distention from overeating and delayed gastric emptying secondary to the increased ingestion of fatty foods leads to prolonged periods of postprandial gastric distention with shortening of the sphincter and results in repetitive transient loss of the barrier (Fig. 4.8). A Nissen fundoplication prevents the shortening of the barrier with progressive degrees of gastric distention by diverting the forces produced by gastric wall tension that pull on the gastroesophageal junction (6). The new endoscopic procedures, Endocinch (Bard, USA) and the Plicator (NDO Surgical, USA), attempt to do the same. Similarly, the endoscopic injection of inert materials into the area of the barrier or scarring it with radiofrequency injury attempts to reduce the compliance of the sphincter, making it more resistant to the pull of gastric wall tension.

In advanced reflux disease, permanent loss of sphincter length occurs from inflammatory injury that extends from the mucosa into the muscular layers of the distal esophagus (3). Fletcher et al. (25) showed that in the fasting state, there is a persistent region of high acidity in the area of the gastroesophageal junction and that this region of acidity migrates 2 cm proximally after meals. This migration occurs as a result of distention of the stomach with eating and pulling apart of the distal HPZ or sphincter, allowing the area of high acidity to move proximal to the squamocolumnar junction. This proximal movement exposes the distal esophageal squamous mucosa to acid, with the formation of cardiac mucosa. Cardiac mucosa is an acquired mucosa and results from inflammatory injury of the squamous mucosa in the terminal esophagus (26). The inflammatory process extends into the muscular layer of the esophagus, resulting in muscle cell injury with permanent shortening of the HPZ or sphincter, and a concomitant reduction in the amplitude of the HPZ or barrier pressure (21,27). A defective barrier is recognized

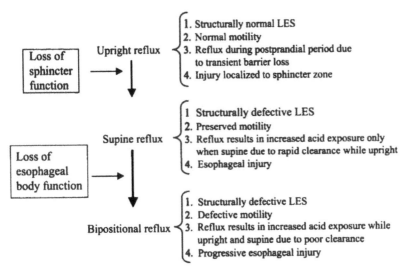

Figure 4.8 Schema of the progression of GERD. Initially esophageal acid exposure occurs only in the upright awake position after meals due to transient losses of the barrier. With inflammatory injury to the LES the barrier becomes permanently defective and an increase in esophageal acid exposure occurs in supine position while gravity and the esophageal body effectively clear the refluxed acid during the day when upright. Inflammatory injury to the esophageal body due to supine acid exposure results in the loss of esophageal body clearance function and increased esophageal acid exposure during the night and day or bipositional reflux.

when the length or pressure of the sphincter measured during the fasting state is below the 2.5th percentile of normal (17). For the clinician, the finding of a permanently defective sphincter has several implications. First, damage to the sphincter is irreversible, consequently patients with a defective sphincter can be difficult to control with medical therapy (28). Surgery is usually required to achieve consistent long-term symptom relief and interrupt the natural history of the disease. It has been shown repeatedly that a laparoscopic Nissen fundoplication can restore the length and pressure of the barrier to normal (29). Secondly, a permanently defective sphincter is commonly associated with reduced contractility and abnormal wave progression of the esophageal body (30). This makes clearance of reflux acid difficult and leads to excessive esophageal exposure to acid. Thirdly, a permanently defective sphincter and the loss of effective esophageal clearance leads to increased esophageal exposure of gastric juice with mucosal injury and the potential for Barrett's metaplasia, as well as repetitive regurgitation, aspiration, and potentially for pulmonary fibrosis (19,31). At this stage of the disease shortening of the esophageal body has usually occurred from the inflammatory injury (20,32). A reduction of as little as 2 cm in esophageal length can place the surgical repair under too much tension, and herniation of the repair into the chest or breakdown of the repair can occur. In this situation an open antireflux procedure with complete mobilization of the thoracic esophagus and, in some situations, performing a gastroplasty procedure to lengthen the esophagus, provides a better long-term outcome (3,32). If the esophageal body has been severely damaged, that is, the contraction amplitude in the lower two-third of the esophagus is globally below 20 mmHg, a stage of disease has been reached where a vagal sparing esophagectomy is the better option than an open antireflux repair.

REFERENCES

1. Allison PR. Reflux esophagitis, sliding hiatal hernia and the anatomy of repair. Surg Gynecol Obstet 1951; 92:419.

2. Carlson MA, Frantzidez CT. Complications and results of primary minimally invasive anti-reflux procedure. A review of 10,735 reported cases. J Am Coll Surg 2001; 193:429–439.

3. DeMeester TR, Peters JH, Bremner CG, Chandrasoma P. Biology of gastroesophageal reflux disease: pathophysiology relating to medical and surgical treatment. Ann Rev Med 1999; 50:469–506.

4. Bonavina L, Evander A., DeMeester TR, Walter B, Cheng SC, Palazzo L, Concannon JL. Length of the distal esophageal sphincter and competency of the cardia. Am J Surg 1986; 151:25–34.

5. Stein HJ, DeMeester TR, Naspetti R, Jamieson J, Perry RE. Three-dimensional imaging of the lower esophageal sphincter in gastroesophageal reflux disease. Ann Surg 1991; 214: 374–384.

6. Mason RJ, Lund RJ, DeMeester TR, Peters JH, Crookes, P, Ritter M, Gadenstätter M, Hagen JA. Nissen fundoplication prevents shortening of the sphincter during gastric distention. Arch Surg 1997; 132:719–726.

7. Pettersson GB, Bombeck CT, Nyhus LM. The lower esophageal sphincter: mechanisms of opening and closure. Surgery 1980; 88:307–314.

8. Dent J. A new technique for continuous sphincter pressure measurement. Gastroenterology 1976; 71:263–267.

9. Ismail T, Bancewicz J, Barlow J. Yield pressure, anatomy of the cardia and gastroesophageal reflux. Br J Surg 1995; 82:943–947.

10. Marchand P. The gastro-oesophageal 'sphincter' and the mechanism of regurgitation. Br J Surg 1955; 42:504–513.

11. Kahrilas PJ, Shi G, Manka M, Joehl RJ. Increased frequency of transient lower esophageal sphincter relaxation induced by gastric distention in reflux patients with hiatal hernia. Gastroenterology 2000; 118:688–695.

12. DeMeester TR, Wernly JA, Bryant GH, Little AG, Skinner DB. Clinical and in vitro analysis of gastroesophageal competence: a study of the principles of antireflux surgery. Am J Surg 1979; 137:39–46.

13. Pellegrini CA, DeMeester TR, Skinner DB. Response of the distal esophageal sphincter to respiratory and positional maneuvers in humans. Surg Forum 1976; 27:380–382.

14. O'Sullivan GC, DeMeester TR, Joelsson BE, Smith RB, Blough RR, Johnson LF, Skinner DB. The interaction of the lower esophageal sphincter pressure and length of sphincter in the abdomen as determinants of gastroesophageal competence. Am J Surg 1982; 143:40–47.

15. Johnson LF, Lin YC, Hong SK. Gastroesophageal dynamics during immersion in water to the neck. J Appl Physiol 1975; 38(3):449–454.

16. DeMeester TR, Wernly JA, Bryant GH, Little AG, Skinner DB. Clinical and in vitro analysis of gastroesophageal competence: a study of the principles of antireflux surgery. Am J Surg 1979; 137:39–46.

17. Zaninotto G, DeMeester TR, Schwizer W, Johansson K-E, Cheng SC. The lower esophageal sphincter in health and disease. Am J Surg 1988; 155:104–111.

18. Stein HJ, Barlow AP, DeMeester TR, Hinder RA. Complications of gastroesophageal reflux disease: role of the lower esophageal sphincter, esophageal acid and acid/alkaline exposure, and duodenogastric reflux. Ann Surg 1992; 216(1):35–43.

19. Tsai P, Peters J, Johnson W, Cohen R, Starnes V. Laparoscopic fundoplication 1 month prior to lung transplantation. Surg Endosc 1996; 10:668–670.

20. Zaninotto G, DeMeester TR, Bremner CG, Smyrk TC, Cheng S-C. Esophageal function in patients with reflux-induced strictures and its relevance to surgical treatment. Ann Thorac Surg 1995; 47:362–370.

21. DeMeester TR, Ireland AP. Gastric pathology as an initiator and potentiator of gastroeso-phageal reflux disease. Dis Esophagus 1997; 10:1–8.

22. Barham CP, Gotley DC, Mills A, Alderson D. Precipitating causes of acid reflux episodes in ambulant patients with gastro-oesophageal reflux disease. Gut 1995; 36:505–510.

23. Bremner RM, Hoeft SF, Costantini M, Crookes PF, Bremner CG, DeMeester TR. Pharyngeal swallowing: the major factor in clearance of esophageal reflux episodes. Ann Surg 1993; 218(3):364–370.

24. Iwakiri K, Kobayashi M, Kotoyari M, Yamada H, Sujiura T, Nakagawa Y. Relationship between postprandial esophageal acid exposure and meal volume and fat content. Dig Dis Sci 1996; 41:926–930.

25. Fletcher J, Wirz A, Young J et al. Unbuffered highly acidic gastric juice exists at the gastro-esophageal junction after a meal. Gastroenterology 2001; 121:775–783.

26. Öberg S, Peters JH, DeMeester TR, Chandrasoma P, Hagen JA, Ireland AP, Ritter MP, Mason RJ, Crookes P, Bremner CG. Inflammation and specialized intestinal metaplasia of cardiac mucosa is a manifestation of early gastroesophageal reflux disease. Ann Surg 1997; 226:322–522.

27. Theisen J, Öberg S, Peters JH et al. Gastro-esophageal reflux disease confined to the sphincter. Dis Esophagus 2001; 14:235–238.

28. Kuster E, Ros E, Toledo-Pimentel V, Pujol A, Bordas JM, GL, Pera C. Predictive factors of the long term outcome in gastro-oesophageal reflux disease: six year follow up of 107 patients. Gut 1994; 35:8–14.

29. Peters JH, DeMeester TR, Crookes P, Öberg S, De Vos Shoop M, Hagen JA, Bremner CG. The treatment of gastroesophageal reflux disease with laparoscopic Nissen fundoplication. Ann Surg 1998; 228:40–50.

30. Singh P, Adamopoulos A, Taylor RH, Colin-Jones DG. Oesophageal motor function before and after healing of oesophagitis. Gut 1992; 33:1590–1596.

31. Stein JH, Eypasch EP, DeMeester TR, Smyrk TC. Circadian esophageal motor function in patients with gastroesophageal reflux disease. Surgery 1990; 108:769–778.

32. Gastal O, Hagen JA, Peters JH, Campos GMR, Hashemi M, Theisen J, Bremner CG, DeMeester TR. Short esophagus: analysis of predictors and clinical implications. Arch Surg 1999; 134:633–638.

7. LOWER ESOPHAGEAL SPHINCTER

There are four methods of recording the LES pressure. They are (1) standard SPT method, (2) rapid pull-through method, (3) motorized pull-through method, and (4) Dent sleeve method.

7.1. Standard Stationary Pull-Through Technique

The motility catheter is passed through the anesthetized nostril and into the stomach. The perfusion system is activated and baseline settings of the gastric pressure are made. The catheter is withdrawn at 1 cm increments until all catheter openings have passed through the sphincter.

The lower esophageal HPZ comprises the LES component and a contribution from the diaphragm. Part of the LES pressure is intra-abdominal and a part is intrathoracic. The RIP, also called the pressure inversion point (PIP), is that point where the upward respiratory deflections change direction to a downward mode. It is the physiological separation point of the intra-abdominal and intrathoracic cavities. The start of the sphincter pressure is measured from the point where the end-expiratory pressure increases >2 mm from the gastric baseline pressure. The sphincter ends at the point where the end-expiratory pressure falls below the gastric baseline pressure.

7.2. Rapid Pull-Through Technique

A continuous manual withdrawal of the recording sensors through the LES is made at an approximate rate of 0.5–1.0 cm/s during a 10–15 s interval of suspended respiration (1). The method avoids recording "artifacts" caused by respiratory LES motion and provides precise end-points for measurement.

Normal value of LES pressure is 24.3 ± 9.5 mmHg compared with 21.1 ± 9.1 mmHg in 12 patients studied by Dodds et al.

7.2.1. Reproducibility of the Rapid Pull-Through Method

Staino and Clouse studied 250 consecutive patients. LES pressure did not differ between two measurements (normals, 25.3 ± 1.0 vs. 26.2 ± 1.0 mmHg, correlation $r = 0.73$).

7.3. Motorized Pull-Through Method

The catheter assembly is pulled through the LES by a mechanized puller attached to the catheter. This is described in detail on p. 72.

7.4. Dent Sleeve

This water-infusion catheter has a specially constructed tip. Water is constantly infused into a 6 cm long membrane that covers the side-holes producing a long pressure sensitive area, which is not affected by displacement of the catheter. Pressure measurements with this system correlate well with the results of the conventional water-perfused method. It is also the only way to measure transient lower esophageal sphincter relaxations (TLESR).

The disadvantage of measuring the LES with this catheter is that the length of the sphincter cannot be assessed and the sleeve constantly measures a shorter duration of relaxation (1).

7.5. Measurement of the LES

The normal HPZ at the hiatus comprises the pressure of the true LES and the pressure due to the diaphragmatic crura. Both components are integrated in the normal LES. The crural component is recognized by high respiratory deflections: the apices of these are sharper than the blunter deflections seen in the true LES.

Sphincter length is measured from the point where the expiratory pressure leaves the intragastric baseline by 2 mmHg (lower level 0), to the point where the expiratory pressure is negative to the baseline (upper border).

Sphincter pressure may be measured by different methods:

1. Mid-expiration at the station with the highest overall pressures. In a study, this method distinguished patients with normal gastroesophageal acid exposure from those with abnormal exposure.
2. End-expiration at the station with the highest overall pressures. This method eliminates the respiratory cycle of the diaphragm.
3. At the RIP, also called the PIP. This method is used in Dr. DeMeester's laboratory. He validated the numbers by *in-vitro* and 24 h pH studies. At the RIP, there is no influence of the respiratory swings. The RIP separates the intrathoracic and intra-abdominal segments, that is, esophagus comprises the intrathoracic and intra-abdominal segments.

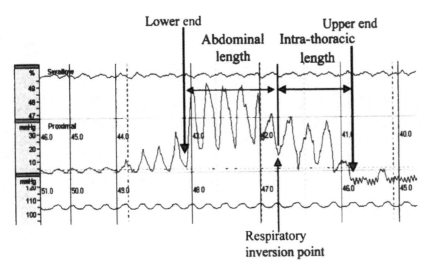

Figure 4.9 A normal LES. The upper end of the LES starts at 41 cm, where the pressure drops to a negative value (intrathoracic). The lower end is at 43 cm, where the pressure rises 2 mm or more above the intragastric pressure baseline.

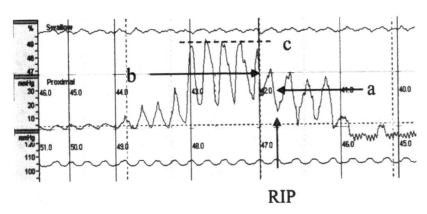

RIP

Figure 4.10 Measurement of the LES pressure. (a) Pressure measured at the mid-respiratory excursion at the RIP. The pressure in this recording is 30 mmHg; (b) Mid-respiratory measurement (40 mmHg); (c) End-inspiratory measurement (48 mmHg); and (d) End-expiratory measurement (20 mmHg).

Table 4.2 Normal LES Parameters in 50 Healthy Volunteers. [After Zaninotto and DeMeester.]

LES measurements	Mean	SD	Median	Maximum	Minimum	Percentile 2.5th	5th
Pressure (mmHg)	14.87	5.14	13.8	25.6	5.2	6.1	8
Abdominal length (cm)	2.18	0.72	2.2	5	0.8	0.89	1.1
Overall length (cm)	3.65	0.68	3.5	5.5	2.4	2.4	2.6

REFERENCES

Aliperti G, Clouse RE. Incomplete esophageal sphincter relaxation in subjects with peristalsis: prevalence and clinical outcome. Am J Gastroenterol 1991; 86(5):609–614.

Allen ML, Dimario A, Robinson M. Premature lower esophageal sphincter closure as a cause of dysphagia. Am J Gastroenterol 1993; 88(9):1377–1380.

Bonavina L, Evander A, DeMeester TR. Length of the distal esophageal sphincter and competency of the cardia. Am J Surg 1986; 151:25–34.

Castell JA, Dalton CB, Castell DO. On-line computer analysis of human lower esophageal sphincter relaxation. Am J Physiol 1988; 255:G794–G799.

Chobanian SJ, Benjamin SB, Castell DO. Characterization of lower esophageal sphincter relaxation in normals. Gastroenterol A Clin Res 1982; 30:723A.

Clouse RE, Staiano A. Contraction abnormalitites of the esophageal body in patients referred for manometry. Dig Dis Sci 1983; 28:784–790.

Clouse RE, Staiano A. Manometric patterns using esophageal body and lower sphincter characteristics. Dig Dis Sci 1992; 37(2):289–295.

DiMarino AJ, Cohen S. Characteristics of lower esophageal sphincter function in symptomatic diffuse esophageal spasm. Gastroenterol 1974; 66:1–5.

Dodds WJ, Hogan WJ, Stef JJ, Miller WM, Lydon SB, Arndorfer RC. A rapid pull-through technique for measuring lower esophageal sphincter pressure. Gastroenterology 1975; 68:437–443.

Fibbe C, Layer P, Keller J, Strate U, Emmerman A, Zornig C. Esophageal motility in reflux disease before and after fundoplication: a prospective randomized clinical and manometric study. Gastroenterology 2001; 121:5–14.

Holloway RH, Penagini R, Ireland AC. Criteria for objective definition of transient lower esophageal sphincter relaxation. Am J Physiol 1995; 265:G128–G133.

Katzka DA, Sidhu M, Castell DO. Hypertensive lower esophageal sphincter pressure and gastroesophageal reflux: an apparent paradox that is not unusual. Am J Gastroenterol 1995; 90(2):280–284.

Nielson IJ, Bremner CG. Lower esophageal resting pressure in achalasia and the response of the sphincter to swallowing and drugs. S Afr Med J 1976; 50:1822–1825.

Penagini R, Picone A, Bianchi PA. Effect of morphine and naloxone on motor response of the esophagus to swallowing and distension. Physiology 1996; 271(4 pt 1):G675–G680.

Richter JE, Wallace C, Castell DO. Esophageal manometry in 95 healthy adult volunteers. Dig Dis Sci 1986; 32:583–592.

Staino A, Clouse RE. Reproducibility of the rapid pull-through technique for categorizing lower esophageal sphincter pressure. Am J Gastroenterol 1991; 86(9):1134–1137.

Stein HJ, Crookes PF, DeMeester TR. Manometric evaluation of lower esophageal sphincter function. Problems Gen Surg 1992; 9:75–90.

Zaninotto G, DeMeester TR. The lower esophageal sphincter in health and disease. Am J Surg 1988; 155:104–111.

8. SLOW MOTORIZED PULL-THROUGH: AN IMPROVED TECHNIQUE TO EVALUATE THE LES (1,2)

Manometric evaluation of the LES is usually performed by the SPT technique, which has the disadvantages of a long performance time and difficulty in obtaining tracings free of swallow-induced artifacts. In contrast, the sMPT technique is quicker and differs from the other commonly used method, the rapid pull-through technique, by allowing the recognition of RIP. The sMPT may demonstrate a hiatal hernia, which is not evident on the SPT study.

The method consists of pulling a catheter with four radial side-holes, at a slow constant rate (1.0 mm/s) using a motor catheter puller (Medtronic), through the LES (Fig. 4.11).

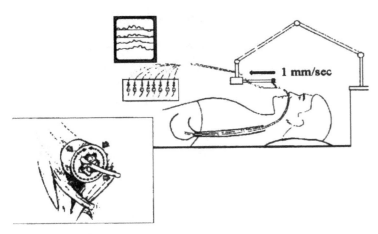

Figure 4.11 How the test is performed. The subject is breathing normally while the motor puller slowly withdraws the catheter across the cardia at a constant speed (1 mm/s). Inset: The four side-holes are located at the same level and oriented at 90 angles. This allows immediate compensation for sphincteral asymmetry and the direct integration of the tracings (e.g., for the three-dimensional reconstruction of the sphincter) (3).

This technique is quick, taking about 1 min for a passage through the sphincter, and well accepted by the patient. It allows high fidelity tracings without swallowing artifacts, even in most difficult patients. The technique also can be performed independent of the operator and lends itself to automated computer analysis.

As the pull-through is performed in a continuous mode, it provides an accurate determination of the sphincter length in millimeter in contrast to the 0.5–1 cm approximation when using the SPT technique. Further, the ease of locating the RIP allows the abdominal length to be calculated. Normal values measured in 41 control subjects are listed in Table 4.3.

Comparison of the motorized to the traditional SPT technique in a group of healthy volunteers and patients with different esophageal disorders revealed a good correlation (4) for pressure (Fig. 4.12) and overall and abdominal length. The technique can be used for the evaluation of both the LES and UES, as well as the anal sphincter.

A basic tenet of esophageal physiology is that the resistance of the LES to the reflux of gastric juice is a function of the integrated effects of pressure exerted over the entire length of the sphincter. The sMPT technique can be used to quantify this function by constructing a three-dimensional computerized image of the sphincter. This is done by plotting the pressure exerted in the four quadrants over the length of the sphincter (Fig. 4.13). The calculated volume of this image reflects the resistance of the LES to the reflux of gastric juice and is called the SPVV (5).

Table 4.3 Normal Ranges of LES Overall Length, Abdominal Length, Mid-cycle Pressure and End-Expiratory Cycle Pressure in 41 Normal Volunteers

	Mean	SD	Median	Min	Max	5th percentile
Overall length (cm)	4.4	1.14	4.4	2.7	6.9	2.7
Abdominal length (cm)	3.0	1.09	2.9	1.1	5.4	1.4
Mid-respiratory pressure (mmHg)	15.8	7.49	16	4.3	37	5.1
End-expiratory pressure (mmHg)	18.8	8.89	18.3	5.3	41.3	6.7

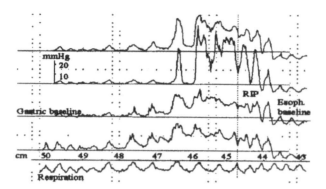

Figure 4.12 Manometric tracings of the LES obtained using the motor pull-through with four side-holes located at the same level and oriented radially at 90° to each other. The RIP is easily identified, and evaluation of the overall and abdominal length of the sphincter is possible. The asymmetry of the LES is evident in that the sphincter is longer in the lower tracing and the pressure is higher in the upper tracing.

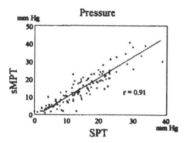

Figure 4.13 Regression analysis of sMPT and SPT methods.

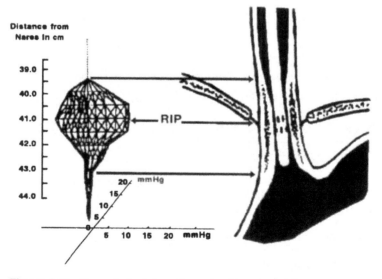

Figure 4.14 Computerized three-dimensional imaging of the LES. A catheter with four to eight radial side-holes is withdrawn through the gastroesophageal junction. For each level, the radially measured pressures are plotted around an axis representing gastric baseline pressure.

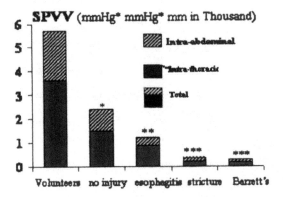

Figure 4.15 Mean total and intra-abdominal SPVV in 50 healthy volunteers and 150 patients with GERD with increased esophageal acid exposure and various degrees of mucosal damage. The P values are given for total and intra-abdominal SPVV. *P < 0.01 vs. volunteers; **P < 0.01 vs. volunteers and GERD patients with no mucosal injury; ***P < 0.01 vs. all other groups.

Figure 4.15 shows that the SPVV are significantly lower in patients with increased esophageal exposure to gastric juice when compared with normal volunteers. Further, the SPVV decreases with increasing severity of mucosal injury. A Nissen antireflux procedure markedly increases the SPVV and as a consequence restores competency (Fig. 4.16). The three-dimensional computerized image of a normal subject and a patient with Barrett's esophagus before and after a Nissen fundoplication are shown in Fig. 4.17.

REFERENCES

1. Costantini M, Bremner RM, Hoeft SF, Crookes PF, DeMeester TR. The slow motorized pull-through: an improved technique to evaluate the lower esophageal sphincter. Gastroenterol 1992; 102:1407.

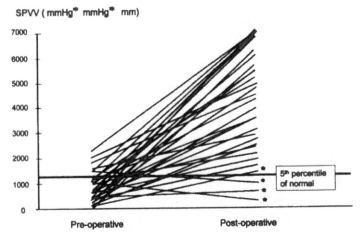

Figure 4.16 Individual preoperative SPVV in 32 patients undergoing antireflux surgery. Asterisk denotes patients with persistent or recurrent reflux. The six preoperative values above the fifth percentile line are six patients who had an isolated abnormality in their abdominal SPVV but a normal total SPVV.

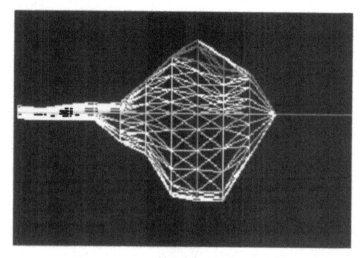

Normal

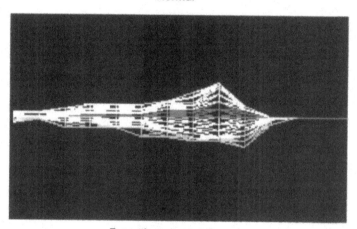

Barrett's pre-operation

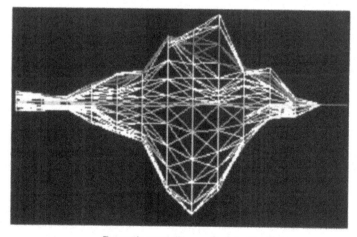

Barrett's post Nissen Fundoplication

Figure 4.17 The three-dimensional sphincter pressure image in a normal volunteer, a patient with Barrett's esophagus, and the same patient after Nissen fundoplication.

2. Campos GMR, Crookes PF, Öberg S, Gastal J, Theisen J, Nigro J, Bremner CG, Peters JH, DeMeester TR. A new standardized method for measurement of the lower esophageal sphincter. Gastroenterol 1998; 114:G3016.

3. Bremner CG, DeMeester TR, Bremner RM, Mason RJ, eds. Esophageal Motility Testing Made Easy. St. Louis, Missouri: Quality Medical Publishing Inc., 2001.

4. Campos GMR, Oberg S, Gastal O, Theisen J, Nigro J, Hagen J, Costantini M, Bremner CG, DeMeester TR, Crookes PF. Manometry of the lower esophageal sphincter. Inter- and Intra-individual variability of slow motorized pull-through versus station pull-through manometry. Dig Dis Sci 2003; 48(6):1057–1061.

5. Stein HJ, DeMeester TR, Naspetti R, Jamieson J, Perry RE. Three-dimensional imaging of the lower esophageal sphincter in gastroesophageal reflux disease. Ann Surg 1999; 214(4):374–384.

9. LES RELAXATION

There is no consensus as to the best method of assessing lower esophageal sphincter relaxation (LESR) despite numerous descriptions. Normal values therefore vary between different laboratories. Residual pressure was preferable to percent of relaxation in Castell's study and was found to be 1.1 ± 0.3 mmHg. Incomplete relaxation of the LES with normal peristalsis is uncommon (1–3). We evaluated 13 previously reported methods in an attempt to identify the best method to standardize this measurement (4).

The following parameters were measured: onset of relaxation, end of relaxation, duration of relaxation, nadir pressure, and peak pressure after relaxation. The methods were ranked based on range, and the spread and variability of values obtained. Nine methods were excluded because the ranges, means, and standard deviations within and between the normals were too wide.

The remaining four techniques of measurement were applied to the recordings of five swallows in each of the 40 volunteers. From these measurements the optimal methods based on small ranges and standard deviations for relaxation were assessed (Fig. 4.18):

1. Duration of relaxation measured from the onset, taken at the peak of the pharyngeal (swallow microphone) recording to the beginning of the upstroke of contraction after the relaxation. Normal: 8.4 s (5th percentile: 6.5 s; 95th percentile: 11.7 s).

2. Minimum residual pressure: The best point at which to measure residual pressure is the time of the upstroke of the peristaltic wave, when recorded in the

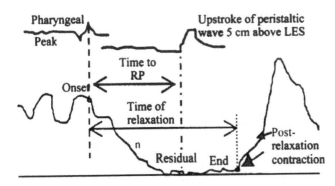

Figure 4.18 Measurement of LESR.

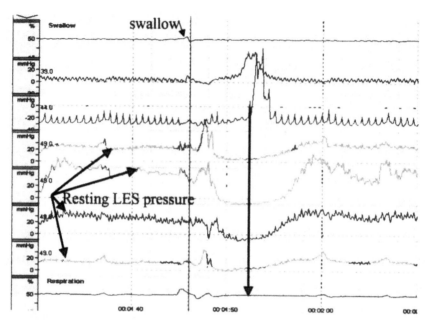

Figure 4.19 Relaxation of the LES following a swallow. Channels 1 and 2 are in the esophagus. Channels 3–6 are recordings of the LES relaxation, all at the same level. Relaxation is complete because the sphincter relaxes to baseline at a point measured from the upstroke of the swallow response 5 cm above.

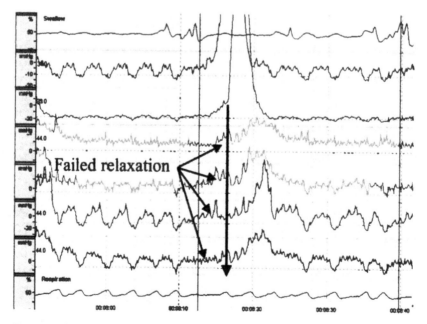

Figure 4.20 Incomplete relaxation of the LES recorded in channels 3–6, all at the same level. The baseline pressure is not reached.

channel 5 cm above the LES. Normal: 3 mmHg (5th percentile: 0.1 mmHg; 95th percentile 7.5 mmHg). Measurements at the nadir are unreliable.

3. Time taken to reach minimum residual pressure. Normal 5.7 s (5th percentile: 4.2 s; 95th percentile: 7.2 s). The ratio of the time to reach minimal residual pressure and the overall duration of relaxation was constant ($R = 0.8$).

REFERENCES

1. Aliperti G, Clouse RE. Incomplete lower esophageal sphincter relaxation with peristalsis: prevalence and clinical outcome. Am J Gastroenterol 1991; 86(5):609–614.
2. Castell JA, Dalton CB, Castell DO. On-line computer analysis of human lower esophageal sphincter relaxation. Am J Physiol 1988; 255:G794–G799.
3. Staino A, Clouse RE. Detection of incomplete lower esophageal sphincter relaxation with conventional point-pressure sensors. Am J Gastroenterol 2001; 96(12):3258–3267.
4. Hamrah P, Bremner CG, Hagen JA, Theisen J, Gastal O, Campos MR, Crookes P, Sillin LF, Peters J, DeMeester TR. Lower esophageal sphincter (LES) relaxation. A standardized method of analysis. Gastroenterol 1999; 116:A1331.

10. TRANSIENT LOWER ESOPHAGEAL SPHINCTER RELAXATION

Relaxation of the LES not induced by a swallow has been described as the main mechanism of gastroesophageal reflux in healthy people and in patients with GERD. Holloway et al. (1) defined TLESRs by:

1. Absence of swallowing for 4 s before to 2 s after the onset of LES relaxation;
2. Relaxation rate of >1 mm/s;
3. Time from onset to complete relaxation of <10 s;
4. Nadir pressure of <2 mmHg.

These relaxations can best be demonstrated by use of the Dent sleeve catheter (2–4). Dent et al. believe that TLESRs are neurally mediated because they do not occur in achalasia or during sleep. They occur especially in the postprandial period and therefore could be related to gastric distension and shortening of the LES. TLESRs are more common in mechanically defective sphincters, and could also be explained by "transient barrier losses" from a failing LES.

REFERENCES

1. Holloway RH, Penagini R, Ireland AC. Criteria for objective definition of transient lower esophageal sphincter relaxation. Am J Physiol 1995; 31:G128–G133.
2. Dent J, Dodds WJ, Friedman RH, Sekiguchi WJ, Hogan WJ, Arndorfer RC, Petrie DJ. Mechanism of gastro-esophageal reflux in recumbent asymptomatic human subjects. J Clin Invest 1980; 65:256–267.
3. Dodds WJ, Dent J, Hogan WJ, Helm JF, Hauser RG, Patel GW, Egide M. Mechanisms of gastro-esophageal reflux in patients with reflux esophagitis. N Engl J Med 1982; 307:1547–1552.
4. Mason RJ, Lund RJ, DeMeester TR, Peters JH, Crookes P, Ritter M, Gadenstatter M, Hagen J. Nissen fundoplication prevents shortening of the sphincter during gastric distension. Arch Surg 1997; 132:719–726.

11. THE MECHANICALLY DEFECTIVE LES

Description

A lower sphincter with measurements that are below the range of normal are likely to be associated with increased esophageal acid exposure. *In vitro* and manometric studies have defined a defective sphincter as follows:

1. LES pressure <6 mmHg (measured at the point of respiratory reversal);
2. Overall length <2 cm;
3. Abdominal length <1 cm.

Table 4.4 Probability of an Abnormal pH Score with Abnormal Sphincter Manometric Results

Sphincter manometric abnormality	Abnormal 24 pH score		
	Total	*n*	(%)
Overall length (<2 cm)	17	13	76
Overall and abdominal length	17	11	65
Pressure (≤6 mmHg)	111	81	73
Abdominal length (<1 cm)	39	27	69
Pressure and overall length	3	2	67
Pressure and abdominal length	43	38	88
Pressure, overall and abdominal length	26	24	92

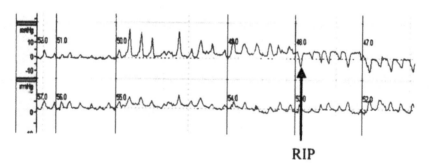

Figure 4.21 Abnormal pressure. The LES pressure in this record was <6 mmHg.

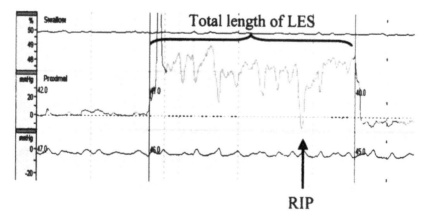

Figure 4.22 Abnormal overall length of the LES. In this record the overall length was only 1 cm.

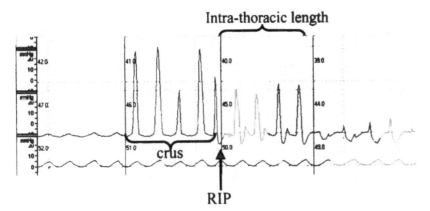

Figure 4.23 Abnormal intra-abdominal length. In this record there is no abdominal length. The respiratory responses before the RIP are from crural impingement only. They do not leave the baseline, indicating that there is no pressure component from the LES.

The probability of an abnormal pH score with abnormal sphincter manometric result is presented in Table 4.4.

12. HYPERTENSIVE LOWER ESOPHAGEAL SPHINCTER

Definition

An HLES has a sphincter pressure, which is above the 95th percentile of normal. The value will differ according to the method used for measurement.

1. Pressure measurement at the end-expiratory pressure level of the highest peaks (Katzka, Sidhu, Castell) (1).
2. According to DeMeester pressure measurement at the point of respiratory reversal (RIP) ≥ 26 mmHg (2).

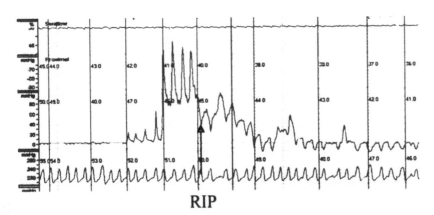

Figure 4.24 Hypertensive lower esophageal sphincter. The pressure exceeds 26 mmHg and the intrathoracic pressure is negative.

The LES may be hypertensive in achalasia (50% cases). The following table gives distinguishing features between the two disorders.

	HLES	Achalasia
Relaxation of LES	usual	Fails or incomplete
Negative intrathoracic pressure	+	Usually negative
Peristaltic swallow responses	+	Never

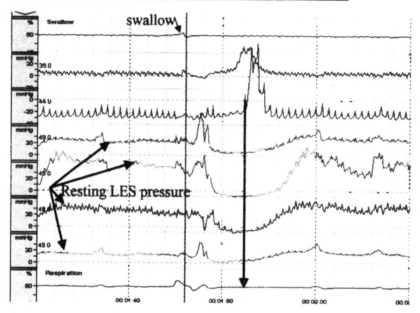

Figure 4.25   The swallow response in a patient with an HLES. Complete relaxation is present.

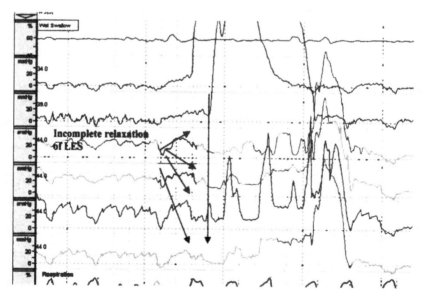

Figure 4.26   The swallow response in a patient with an HLES with incomplete relaxation. Note the increased bolus pressure measured in the body contraction 5 cm above the LES (see bolus pressure on page 104).

12.1.   HLES with a Pressurized Esophagus (see Section 41.5)

This may be a form of atypical achalasia. It is possible that when the outflow obstruction is less severe, peristalsis may be preserved.

This phenomenon may explain why an achalasia pattern is sometimes seen after a tight Nissen fundoplication operation, but not when a "floppy" Nissen operation is accomplished.

13.   LES IN ACHALASIA (3–6)

The cause of the changes in achalasia are unknown but are associated with an absence of the neurotransmitters, nitric oxide and vasopressin.

Features

1. Hypertensive in $\pm 50\%$ cases.
2. Relaxation is either absent, incomplete or of a short duration.
3. The proximal pressure drop is usually, but not always, positive to intragastric pressure.

Note: The features of the LES in achalasia are not always diagnostic. The LES pressure is not hypertensive in 50% of cases, relaxation may take place but is usually abnormal and the esophagus may not be pressurized.

The most important diagnostic feature in achalasia is seen in the body where the swallow responses are simultaneous, that is, the absence of peristalsis.

REFERENCES

1. Katzka DA, Sidhu M, Castell DO. Hypertensive lower esophageal sphincter and gastroesophageal reflux; an apparent paradox that is not unusual. Am J Gastroenterology 1995; 90:280–284.
2. Stein HJ, Crookes PF, DeMeester TR. Manometric evaluation of lower esophageal sphincter function. Probl Gen Surg 1992; 9:75–90.
3. Sanderson DR, Ellis FH, Schlegel JF, Olsen AM. Syndrome of vigorous achalasia: clinical and physiologic observations. Dis Chest 1967; 52:508–517.
4. Goldberg SP, Burrell M, Fette GG, Vos C, Traube M. Classic and vigorous achalasia: a comparison of manometric, radiographic and clinical findings. Gastroenterology 1991; 101:743–748.

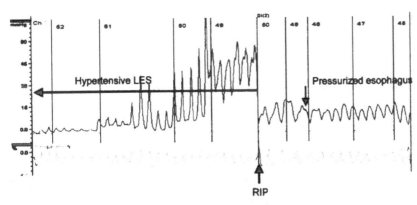

Figure 4.27   The LES in achalasia. Note the high pressure and the positive intrathoracic pressure ("pressurized esophagus").

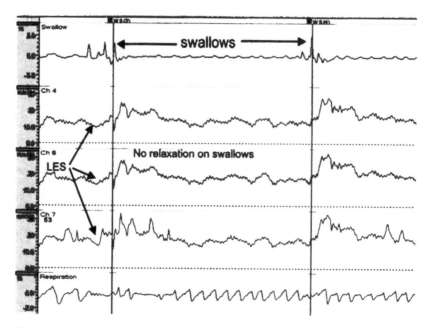

Figure 4.28 Swallow responses in achalasia. The sphincter fails to relax. Channels 5–8 are at the same level and record the high pressure in the LES.

5.   Nielsen IJ, Bremner CG. Lower esophageal sphincter resting pressures in achalasia and the response of the sphincter to swallowing and drugs. S Afr Med J 1976; 50:1822–1825.
6.   Katz PO, Richter JE, Cowan R, Castell DO. Apparent complete lower esophageal sphincter relaxation in achalasia. Gastroenterology 1986; 90(4):978–983.

14. CRURAL PATTERN

The respiratory peaks detected by a perfused catheter system are sharp pointed when measured at the crura and are blunt-pointed when measured in the LES. Peak pressures at the diaphragm occur at end-inspiration and correspond with the peak diaphragmatic

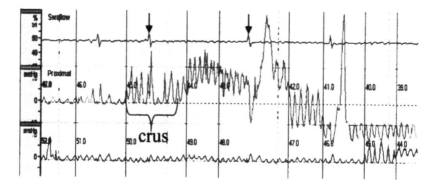

Figure 4.29 Effect of a swallow on the crural pressure. During swallowing there is a transient breath-holding and the respiratory excursion at the crura will stop temporarily until the next breath is taken. The LES drops in response to a swallow because of relaxation of the sphincter.

electromyogram in the experimental model (1). The LES pressure during apnea is equal to end-expiratory pressure during spontaneous respiration.

REFERENCE

1. Boyle JT, Altschuler SM, Todd NE, Tuchman DN, Pack AI, Cohen S. Role of the diaphragm in the genesis of lower esophageal sphincter pressures in the cat. Gastroenterology 1985; 88:723–730.

15. HIATAL HERNIA

Type I hernia. The LES is displaced into the chest. This is the commonest type of hernia.

Type II hernia. This is a true paraesophageal hernia, which is very uncommon. The LES is not displaced. Part or all of the fundus of the stomach displaces into the chest.

Type III hernia. This is the usual type of "paraesophageal" hernia. The LES is displaced into the chest and part of the fundus is also displaced.

Type IV hernia. The LES and whole stomach are displaced into the chest. The hiatal defect is usually large and abdominal viscera (small and large bowel, spleen) also commonly herniate into the chest.

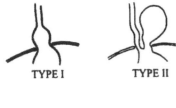

TYPE I   TYPE II

TYPE III   TYPE IV
          (intrathoracic stomach)

Figure 4.30   Types of hiatal hernia.

16. TYPE I HERNIA

Description

The LES is displaced into the chest.

Manometric features

1. Major
      Double hump (two peaks of pressure) (1–3)
      Double respiratory reversal (1)

      Increased length (76 cm) (2)

      Plateau (1,4). The pressure in the plateau is variable.

      Absence of intra-abdominal length of the LES (intrathoracic RIP)

      Indications of sliding

      Excessive pressure swings

      Short esophagus

2. Minor

      Altered motor action with swallowing

         – Post relaxation

         – Excessive contraction (6)

      Hypotonic high-pressure zone (HPZ) (7)

      Hypertonic HPZ

Double respiratory reversal is seen in 52.5%; double hump in 49%; increased length in 55.4%; plateau in 21% (8).

REFERENCES

1. Code CF, Kelley MC, Schlegel JF, Olsen AM. Detection of hiatal hernia during esophageal motility tests. Gastroenterology 1962; 43:521–531.
2. Greenwood RK, Schlegel JF, Helm WJ, Code CF. Pressure and potential difference characteristics of surgically created hiatal hernia. Gastroenterology 1965; 48:602–611.
3. Atkinson M, Edwards DA, Honour AJ, Rowlands EN. The oesophago-gastric sphincter in hiatus hernia. Lancet 1957; 2:1138–1142.
4. Kelley ML. The clinical application of esophageal motility tests. Ann Int Med 1963; 59:338–350.
5. Vela AR, Balart LA. The clinical value of esophageal intraluminal manometry. Am Surg. 1968; 34:39–47.
6. Moroz SP, Espinoza J, Cumming WA, Diamant NE. Lower esophageal sphincter function in children with and without gastroesophageal reflux. Gastroenterology 1976; 71:236.
7. Vantrappen G, Liemer MD, Ikeya J, Texter EC, Baborka CJ. Simultaneous fluorocine-matography and intraluminal pressure measurements in the study of esophageal motility. Gastroenterology 1958; 35:592.
8. Henderson RD. Esophageal Manometry in Clinical Investigation. New York: Praeger, 1983: 50–75.

17. SLIDING HIATAL HERNIA

As the LES displaces upward it moves away from the hiatus, so that the two components of the HPZ are separated. This results in "two pressure humps," which usually signify the presence of a hiatal hernia. The space between the humps is named the "plateau." The length of the plateau corresponds to the length of the hernia.

Note: A hiatal hernia seen radiologically may have reduced during the supine position taken during the manometry test and may not be evident on the recording. The motorized pull-through method may detect a hernia not seen on the pull-through method. If the crural hiatus is lax and wide open, manometry may not detect any crural pressure. A hiatal hernia in such circumstances would be recorded as a plateau with a single pressure from the LES. Likewise, the LES pressure may be very poor resulting in a single pressure recording from the crura and a plateau.

17.1. Cartoon Description of the Evolution of a Sliding Hiatal Hernia

In normal subjects the squamocolumnar junction is 0.5 cm below the hiatus, and the gastroesophageal junction HPZ is 1.1 cm distal to that point. As the LES moves upwards into the chest, the crural component of the LES becomes separated from the composite HPZ. In patients with a hiatal hernia the HPZ, therefore, has two discrete segments, one proximal to the squamocolumnar junction and one distal due to the compression of the stomach within the hiatal canal (1) (Fig. 4.31).

(a) A normal lower esophageal HPZ is a composite of the intrinsic LES pressure and the pressure exerted by the crus of the diaphragm. The high sharper peaks represent the crural component, and are normally at the proximal end of the HPZ.

(b) In the genesis of a hiatal hernia the two components of the HPZ start to separate. The crural component is now displacing to the caudal end of the HPZ.

(c) The separation is complete and the pressure profile of the crus assumes a distinctive character, starting at the baseline and with sharper peaks than seen in the pressure profile of the intrinsic LES.

(d) As the separation continues, two distinct pressure profiles become evident— The "double hump," which is typical of a sliding hiatal hernia.

(e) The separation has continued, and the two "humps" are separated by a plateau of lower pressure.

(f) In this cartoon of a sliding hiatal hernia, there is no distinct pressure profile of the hiatus, presumably because the hiatus is widely open so that it does not compress the stomach at that point.

(g) In this cartoon, the hiatal pressure is obvious, but there is a very low pressure from the intrinsic sphincter.

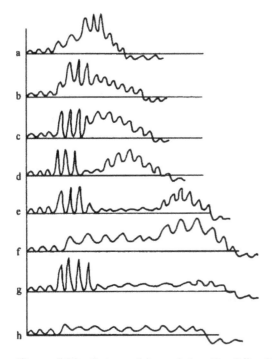

Figure 4.31 Cartoon of the evolution of a sliding hiatal hernia.

(h) In this cartoon, there is no pressure detectable from the crus, but a very poor pressure from the intrinsic LES. Only the presence of a plateau gives evidence of a hiatal hernia.

Note: The RIP is not depicted in these cartoons, and will also give assistance in the recognition of a displaced LES.

Cuomo et al. (2) described five manometric profiles associated with hiatal hernia. Absence of peak pressures at the level of the diaphragmatic hiatus and the LES (flat profile) represented a major impairment of the esophagogastric junction, and these patients had an increased number of reflux episodes. A double-peaked profile signified displacement of the LES and diaphragmatic crura without functional impairment.

REFERENCES

1. Kahrilis PJ, Lin S, Chen J, Manka M. The effect of hiatus hernia on gastro-esophageal junction pressure. Gut 1999; 44:476–482.
2. Cuomo R, Grasso R, Sarnelli G, Bruzzese D, Bottiglieri ME, Alfieri M, Sifrim D, Budillou G. Role of diaphragmatic crura and lower esophageal sphincter in gastro-esophageal reflux disease: manometric and pH-metric study of small hiatal hernia. Dig Dis Sci 2001; 46(12):2687–2694.

17.2. Motility Records Demonstrating Different Phases in the Development of a Sliding Hiatal Hernia

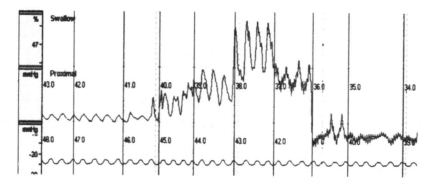

Figure 4.32 A normal LES. The crus is at the upper end of the HPZ. The LES is mostly intra-abdominal.

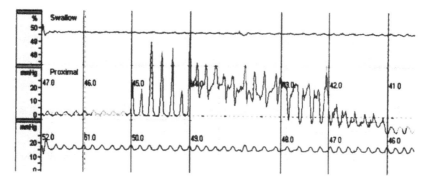

Figure 4.33 The crural component is at the lowermost position of the HPZ (44–45 cm).

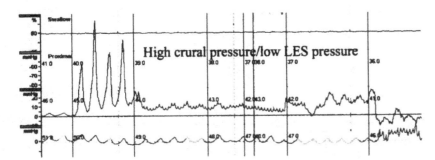

Figure 4.34 The LES component of the HPZ has separated from the crural position, resulting in a hiatal hernia with a double hump and an intervening plateau of pressure, which is 2 cm in length (37–39 cm). This represents a small hiatal hernia.

17.3. Different Motility Patterns of Sliding Hiatal Hernias

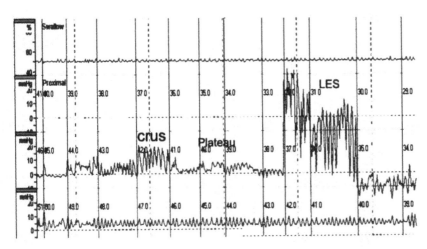

Figure 4.35 A double hump with a low crural pressure and a high LES pressure.

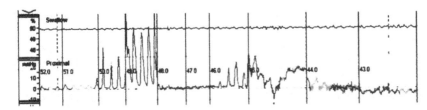

Figure 4.36 A double hump with a high crural pressure and a low LES pressure.

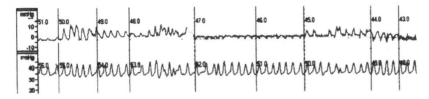

Figure 4.37 A double hump with low crural and LES pressures.

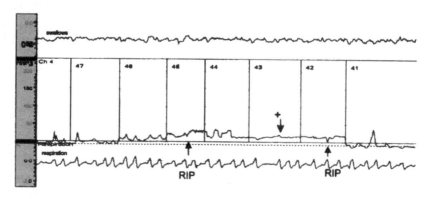

Figure 4.38 No crural or LES pressure. The presence of a plateau may be the only feature suggesting a hiatal hernia.

Note: Significantly higher crural pressures in patients with supine reflux may act as a mechanical barrier and give protection against the unfolding of the LES during the postprandial and upright periods. Higher crural–sphincter pressure gradients and larger sized hiatal hernias in patients with supine reflux results in pressurization of the hernia sac and subsequent reflux when these patients are in the supine position (1).

REFERENCE

1. Banki F, Mason RJ, Hagen JA, Bremner CG, Streets CG, Peters JH, DeMeester TR. The crura and crura-sphincter pressure dynamics in patients with isolated upright and isolated supine reflux. Am Surg 2001; 67:1–7.

18. DOUBLE RESPIRATORY REVERSAL

A double respiratory reversal is a feature seen in some recordings of hiatal hernia. The genesis of such a change in the respiratory reversal is not clearly understood. A hernia into the thoracic cavity will be covered by a layer of peritoneum carried upwards into the chest, resulting in a cavity which is still in continuity with the positive pressure within the abdomen. However, this cavity may be temporarily obliterated when the stomach is impacted into the hiatal ring so that the pressure within the cavity reverts to the negative intrathoracic pressure. This would also explain the repeated reversals, which are also present in some tracings. The detection of a double reversal may be helpful in the diagnosis especially when a double hump is not evident.

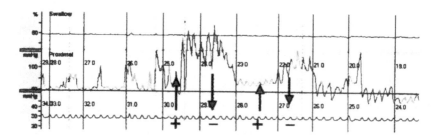

Figure 4.39 A SPT recording of the LES. A changing respiratory reversal is demonstrated.

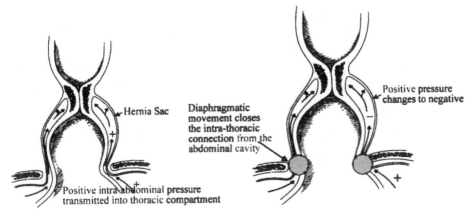

Figure 4.40 Genesis of a changing respiratory reversal.

19. INTRATHORACIC STOMACH

Description

The whole stomach and LES are within the thoracic cavity.

Manometric features

1. Respiratory deflections are negative in all channels at the outset.
2. The LES is well within the thorax.
3. The esophagus is shortened.

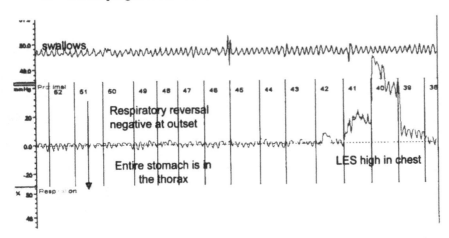

Figure 4.41 Manometric study of an intrathoracic stomach. The respiratory reversal is negative from the outset, showing that the stomach is in the thorax. The LES is high in the chest (short esophagus).

20. THE PLATEAU PRESSURE

The plateau pressure is variable (2–18 mmHg; mean 8 mmHg as measured in 25 patients) (1). A major determinant of the plateau pressure is the LES competency. Larger hernias tend to have a decreased plateau pressure which may be related to the increased capacity of the large hernia, and the greater volume required to pressurize the hernia.

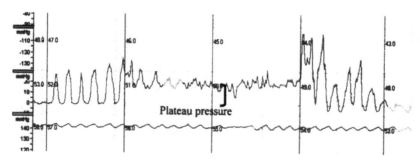

Figure 4.42 A high plateau pressure in a 2 cm hiatal hernia.

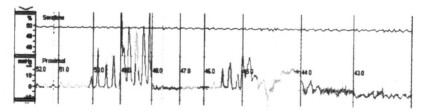

Figure 4.43 A low plateau pressure.

REFERENCE

1. Balaji NS, Wajed S, Bremner CG, Streets C et al. The significance of the plateau pressure in a hiatal hernia noted on esophageal manometry. Gastroenterology 2001; 120(suppl.):2187Abst.

21. ESOPHAGEAL BODY

The esophageal body length is measured from the lower border of the UES to the upper border of the UES. The length varies with the height of the person as demonstrated in the diagram (Fig. 4.44) (1,2). At rest, the end-expiratory pressure in the body is -3 to -5 mmHg relative to intragastric pressure. Following a swallow there is a progressive

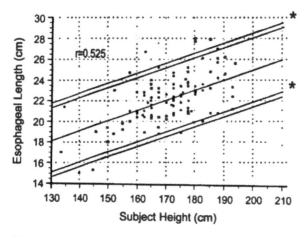

Figure 4.44 Variation of esophageal length with height.

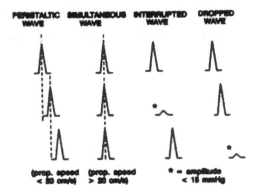

Figure 4.45 Esophageal contraction responses ("waves") are classified into peristaltic, simultaneous, interrupted, and dropped sequences.

peristaltic pressure response. The pressure of each response is measured at the peak of pressure and the duration of the response is measured from the onset of the upstroke to the return point at the baseline. The duration of the contraction, the slope of the contraction wave, and the propagation time can be calculated from these recordings.

22. NORMAL SWALLOW RESPONSES

In our laboratory the first recording site is located 1 cm below the lower border of the UES and the other recording sites are therefore at 6, 11, 16, and 21 cm below the UES. This

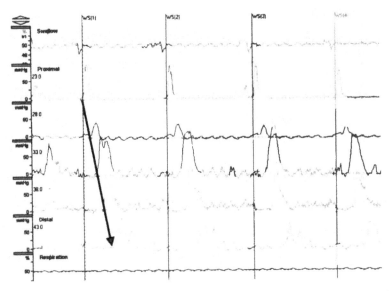

Figure 4.46 Normal swallow responses to four swallows in the esophageal body. The pressure sensors are positioned in the esophagus at 5 cm intervals. Note that there is a progressive peristaltic contraction from above downwards. The responses in channel 2 are usually of a lower amplitude than in the subsequent channels. (The upper esophageal muscle is striated.) WS = wet swallow. The software programme allows a graphic display of the amplitude, duration, propagation, and progression of the cumulated swallow responses, as shown in the four graphs (below right). The hatched boxes depict the 5th and 95th percentiles of normal.

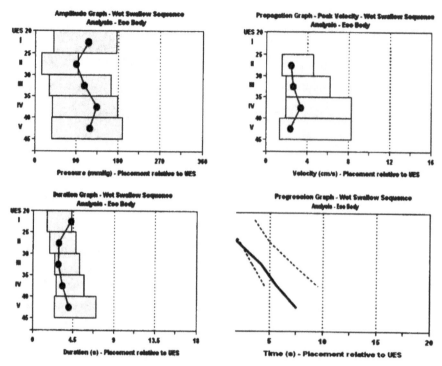

Figure 4.47 A graphic display of normal amplitudes, duration of contractions, and wave progression. Areas I to V represent 5 cm esophageal segments according to the spacing of the open-tips on the catheter assembly. Each box represents the 5th and 95th percentiles of normal and the 2.5th and 7.5th percentiles of normal. Normal peristaltic responses to three swallows.

allows a standard evaluation of the esophageal body contractility. Some laboratories place the open-tip positions referenced to the LES.

Wet swallow responses to a 5 cc water bolus are more reliable than the responses from a dry swallow.

REFERENCES

1. Bremner RM, Crookes PF, Costantini M, DeMeester TR, Peters JH. The relationship of esophageal length to hiatal hernia in gastroesophageal reflux disease (GERD). Gastroenterology 1992; 103(4):A53.
2. Bremner CG. Lower esophageal sphincter position in relation to patients' height. S Afr J Surg 1975; 13:76.

23. DEGLUTITIVE INHIBITION

Every pharyngeal swallow is normally followed by a peristaltic esophageal contraction. During rapid successive swallowing, however, esophageal activity is inhibited until the conclusion of the last swallow. This phenomenon is called "deglututive inhibition," and allows rapid eating and drinking without interference of food or liquid passage through the esophagus (Fig 4.48). Swallow responses are inhibited by repetitive swallowing (1,2). The clinician reading the motility record must be aware of this phenomenon so as to avoid misinterpretation of the poor responses following these swallows.

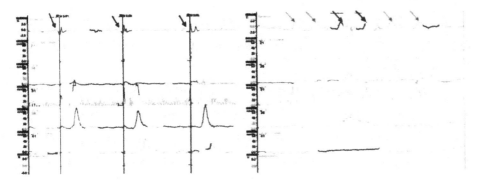

Figure 4.48 The same patient who was asked to swallow repetitively. Note how the peristalsis is inhibited giving a pseudo-appearance of ineffective esophageal motility.

Table 4.5 Normal Swallow Values: Medians (5th and 95th Percentiles)

		Wet swallows	Dry swallows
Amplitude (mmHg)			
	Level I	88 [40–177]	74 [26–154]
	Level II	40 [14–94]	28 [14–74]
	Level III	76 [30–164]	52 [26–142]
	Level IV	93 [38–180]	61 [20–148]
	Level V	93 [36–190]	78 [22–172]
Duration (s)			
	Level I	2.3 [1.5–4.3]	2.3 [1.4–3.9]*
	Level II	3.1 [1.8–4.8]	2.8 [1.0–4.5]
	Level III	3.3 [2.4–5.2]	3.1 [1.8–4.6]
	Level IV	3.6 [2.6–5.7]	3.4 [2.0–5.6]
	Level V	3.7 [2.4–7.0]	3.6 [2.4–6.4]*
Slope (mmHg/s)			
	Level I	99 [22–222]	72 [25–153]
	Level II	30 [9–61]	22 [6–61]
	Level III	52 [20–117]	40 [14–96]
	Level IV	66 [25–120]	45 [14–102]
	Level V	62 [23–120]	47 [16–104]
Propagation speed (cm/s)			
	Level I	2.4 [1.5–4.6]	2.8 [1.6–6.2]
	Level II–III	2.8 [1.9–6.2]	3.1 [1.9–8.3]
	Level III–IV	3.8 [1.9–8.3]	4.5 [1.8–8.3]
	Level IV–V	2.6 [1.3–8.3]	3.5 [1.7–12]
	Level I–IV	2.9 [2.2–3.7]	3.3 [2.3–4.4]
	Level I–V	2.9 [2.1–4]	3.4 [2.2–5]

*All parameters (except those indicated by asterisk) differ between dry and wet swallows ($p < 0.05$, Wilcoxon signed–rank test).

Note: The values and ranges are similar to the results of studies on 95 healthy volunteers reported by Richter JE, Wu WC, Johns DN, Blackwell JN, Nelson JL, Castell JA, Castell DO. Esophageal manometry in 95 healthy adult volunteers. Dig Dis Sci 1987; 32:583–592.

Source: Contantini M, Bremner RM, Hoeft SF, Crookes PF, DeMeester TR. Normal esophageal motor function: a manometric study of 136 healthy subjects. Gastroenterology 1992; 103:A1407.

REFERENCES

1. Ask P, Tibbling L. Effect of time interval between swallows on esophageal peristalsis. Am J Physiol 1980; 238:G485.
2. Vanek AW, Diamant NE. Responses of the human esophagus to paired swallows. Gastroenterology 1987; 92:643.

24. ACHALASIA

Description

Achalasia is a motility disorder of the esophagus characterized by an outflow obstruction caused by inadequate relaxation of the LES, a pressurized and a dilated hypomotile esophagus with simultaneous (mirror-image) swallow responses. The inadequate relaxation of the LES is due to an absence of the neurotransmitters, nitric oxide and vasoactive intestinal polypeptide. Experimental models suggest that the motility abnormalities in the esophagus are secondary to the outflow obstruction. The term "vigorous achalasia" has been used to describe swallow responses which are either of normal or of high amplitude, and which are often repetitive in character. The classification into two types has no clinical significance.

Motility Features

- LES
  Resting pressure is frequently high;
  Swallow responses: relaxation is incomplete (residual pressure >5 mmHg), premature or short-lived (3). Occasionally relaxation may be complete (4).

- Body of esophagus
  Resting pressure is elevated (5–10 mmHg);
  Swallow responses are simultaneous and hypomotile.
- Cricopharyngeal sphincter
  Resting pressure is normal;
  Swallow responses are normal.

24.1. Absence of Peristalsis is the Most Important Diagnostic Feature

The swallow responses are "mirror image" simultaneous responses, and usually have a low amplitude. Swallow responses that are simultaneous and have amplitudes in the normal range also occur, and such a motility pattern has been called vigorous achalasia. Vigorous achalasia does not have any clinical significance and is treated by the same methods as for the usual pattern of achalasia.

24.2 Atypical Achalasia

Variants of the manometric pattern of achalasia occur occasionally and may confuse the clinician. Additional clinical data must then be used to support the diagnosis, for example, radiological evidence of stasis, a bird-beak appearance at the gastroesophageal junction and the absence of air bubble in the stomach. Tatum et al. (1) identified four distinct variants: (a) the presence of high amplitude body contractions; (b) a short segment of esophageal body aperistalsis; (c) retained complete deglutitive LES relaxation; and (d) intact transient LES relaxation.

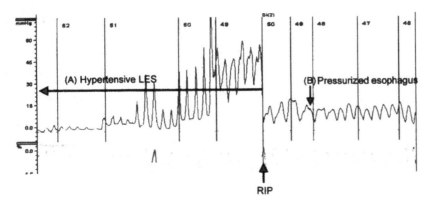

Figure 4.49   (A) A high resting LES pressure. (B) A positive intrathoracic esophageal pressure.

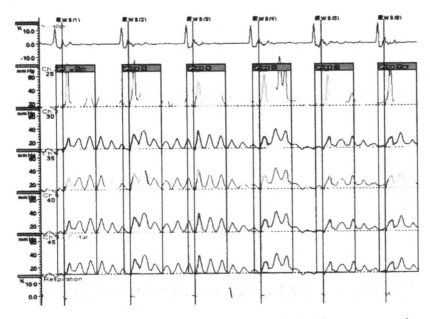

Figure 4.50   Swallowing response in the esophageal body. The responses are hypomotile and simultaneous (mirror image waves secondary to a common cavity).

REFERENCE

1. Tatum HI, Shi G, Sang Q, Joehl RJ, Kahrilis PJ. Manometric heterogeneity in patients with idiopathic achalasia. Gastroenterology 2001; 120(4):789–798.

25. CHAGAS' DISEASE

Chagas' disease results in a progressive loss of the myenteric plexus secondary to infection with *Trypanosome cruzi*.

Manometric features

1. The esophageal manometric features of Chagas' disease are identical to those of achalasia. If the patient comes from an endemic area (Brazil), has any cardiac, colonic, or urinary symptoms, serologic tests for Chagas' should be done.

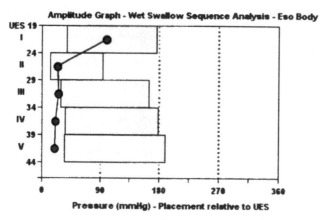

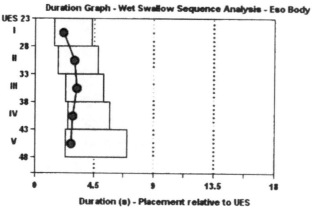

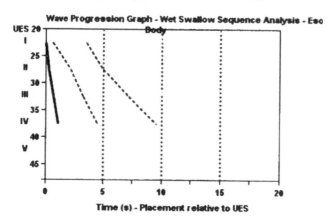

Figure 4.51 Graphic display of the body motility in achalasia. (Top) Amplitude of contractions is below the 5th percentile of normal. (Middle) The duration of the responses is within normal limits. (Bottom) Wave progression. There is no wave progression because the responses are simultaneous.

26. DIFFUSE (DISTAL) ESOPHAGEAL SPASM

Definition

This is a clinical syndrome characterized by symptoms of substernal pain or dysphagia or both, the radiographic appearance of localized nonprogressive waves (tertiary contractions), and an increased incidence of nonperistaltic contractions recorded by intraluminal manometry (1). Because the abnormal contractions are usually seen in the distal esophagus, Dr Castell has suggested that the term *distal esophageal spasm* is more appropriate. This is an uncommon condition, accounting for 3–10% of all motility abnormalities (2,3).

Manometric features

1. Simultaneous contractions in >20% of wet swallows, intermixed with normal peristalsis (4). This is the most consistent finding.
2. Distal esophageal contractions may be high (>110 mmHg), in which case the patient is more likely to have chest pain or low (0.74 mmHg), which is more likely to result in dysphagia (5).
3. Contractions may be repetitive (less than 3 peaks), prolonged (6) or retrograde (7,8).

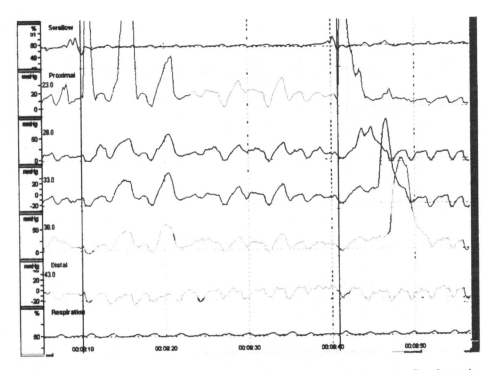

Figure 4.52 Diffuse esophageal spasm. Body motility in a patient who has noncardiac chest pain. Simultaneous responses are presented in all channels of the wet swallow responses after the first swallow. The second swallow is followed by peristaltic responses.

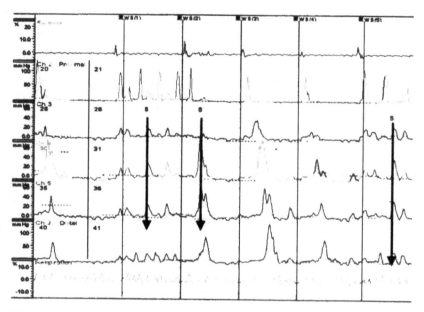

Figure 4.53 Diffuse esophageal spasm. Body motility in a patient who had dysphagia unrelated to a stricture or gastroesophageal reflux. Simultaneous responses are noted after the first, second, and fifth wet swallows. Responses are peristaltic after the third and fourth swallows.

REFERENCES

1. Fleshler B. Diffuse esophageal spasm. Gastroenterology 1967; 52:559.
2. Dalton CB et al. Diffuse esophageal spasm (DES): a rare motility disorder not characterized by high contractile amplitudes. Dig Dis Sci 1991; 36:1025.
3. Katz PO et al. Esophageal testing of patients with non-cardiac chest pain and/or dysphagia. Results of a three year experience with 1161 patients. Ann Int Med 1987; 106:593.
4. Richter JE, Castell DO. Diffuse esophageal spasm: an-appraisal. Ann Int Med 1987; 32:95.
5. Allen M, DiMarino AJ. Manometric diagnosis of diffuse esophageal spasm. Dig Dis Sci 1996; 41:1346.
6. Eypasch EP, DeMeester TR, Klingman RR, Stein HJ. Physiological assessment and surgical management of diffuse esophageal spasm. J Thorac Cardiovasc Surg 1992; 104:859–868.
7. Dalton CB, Castell CO, Hensen EG, Wu WC, Richter JE. Diffuse esophageal spasm. A rare motility disorder not characterized by high amplitude contractions. Dig Dis Sci 1991; 36:1025–1028.
8. Campo S, Traube M. Lower esophageal sphincter dysfunction in diffuse esophageal spasm. Am J Gastroenterol 1989; 84:928.

27. HYPERCONTRACTILE (NUTCRACKER ESOPHAGUS)

Definition

These are high amplitude peristaltic contractions in a patient who has noncardiac chest pain, or rarely, dysphagia (1).

Manometric features

1. Distal esophageal pressures >180 mmHg (mean of 10 swallows) (2).
2. Prolonged duration contractions with normal amplitude (3).

Note: Long-term follow-up with repeated manometric studies revealed a consistency of the diagnosis in 54% of patients (4).

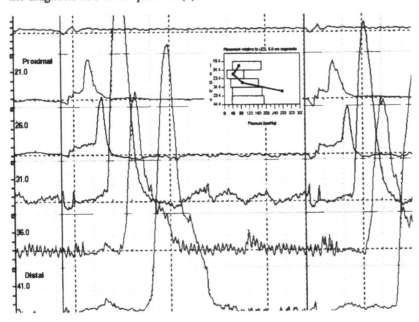

Figure 4.54 There are hypercontractile responses in channels 3, 4, and 5. The *insert* is a graphic display of pressures which are outside of the 95th percentile of normal.

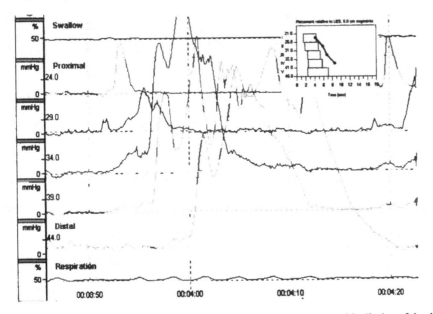

Figure 4.55 Prolonged duration of contractions. The *insert* is a graphic display of the duration of the contractions.

102   **Bremner et al.**

REFERENCES

1. Brand DL, Martin D, Pope CE. Esophageal manometry in patients with angina type chest pain. Am J Dig Dis 1977; 23:300.
2. Benjamin SB, Castell DO. The "nutcracker esophagus" and the spectrum of esophageal motor disorders. Curr Concepts Gastroenterol 1980; 5:3.
3. Herrington JP, Burns TW, Balart LA. Chest pain and dysphagia in patients with prolonged peristaltic contractile duration in the esophagus. Dig Dis Sci 1984; 29:134.
4. Dalton CB, Castell DO, Richter JE. The changing face of the nutcracker esophagus. Am J Gastroenterol 1988; 83:623.

28. VASCULAR ARTIFACTS

The heart, aorta, or abnormal subclavian artery (dysphagia lusoria) may abut on the esophagus and give characteristic pressure profiles. These pressure profiles do not follow the respiratory swings, which are seen in normal motility patterns, but have rapid fluctuations mimicking the heart rate. The baseline of these pressure swings are usually positive by a few millimeters of mercury. Cardiac artifacts are usually above the LES zone, and impressions from the aorta or abnormal subclavian artery are at a higher level. Occasionally a cardiac artifact may be seen at the upper limit of the LES, and care must be taken not to include the pressure rise in the evaluation of the length of the LES.

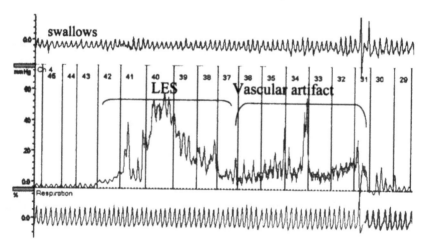

Figure 4.56 A vascular artifact abutting on the lower esophageal sphincter. This may interfere with the correct measurement of the length of the sphincter.

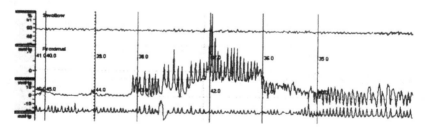

Figure 4.57 A manometric recording of a vascular pressure rise high in the esophagus. This could be due to the heart, aorta, or a vascular abnormality.

29. DYSPHAGIA LUSORIA (FROM LATIN LUSUS NATURAE: A SPORT OF NATURE)

Definition

Dysphagia lusoria is a compression by the right subclavian artery passing behind the esophagus. Several major vascular structures close to the esophagus may press on it and cause dysphagia. An aberrant right subclavian artery is the most common anomaly occurring in 0.6–1.8% of subjects (1–3). The anomaly may be asymptomatic, but symptoms may be present at birth. The barium swallow may show an oblique band 1–2 cm

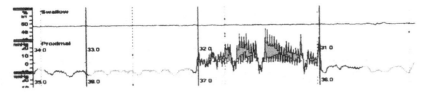

Figure 4.58 A vascular impression which is at a high level in the esophagus (31 cm from the nares) due to a retroesophageal subclavian artery (dysphagia lusoria).

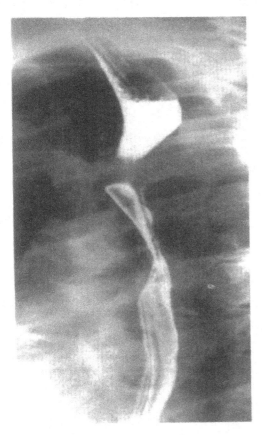

Figure 4.59 A barium swallow examination showing compression of the upper esophagus with dilatation and stasis above the compressed segment.

wide compressing the esophagus at a level which may vary between C6 and T4, but is usually at the level of the tracheal bifurcation.

Manometric feature

1. A pressure rise of about 10 mmHg in the upper esophagus usually 23–25 cm from the incisor teeth.

REFERENCES

1. Janssen M, Baggen MG, Veen HF, Smout AJ, Bekkers JA, Jonkman JG, Owendijk RJ. Dysphagia lusoria: clinical aspects, manometric findings, diagnosis and therapy. Am J Gastroenterol 2000; 95:1411–1416.
2. Nguyen P, Gideon RM, Castell DO. Dysphagia lusoria in the adult: associated esophageal manometric findings and diagnostic use of scanning techniques. Am J Gastroenterol 1994; 89:620–623.
3. Berenzweig H, Baue AE, McCallum RW. Dysphagia lusoria: report of a case and review of diagnostic and surgical approach. Dig Dis Sci 1980; 25:630–636.

30. RAMP INTRABOLUS PRESSURE (1,2)

Following a liquid swallow three pressure responses may be seen.

1. A filling bolus pressure which appears simultaneously at each level in the esophagus. This pressure rise is due to the sudden filling of the esophagus with liquid and is not always present;

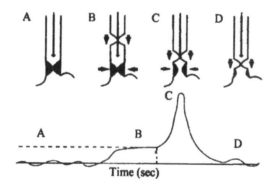

Time (sec)

Figure 4.60 "A" represents the resting intraesophageal pressure: only the background respiratory fluctuations are recorded. "B" shows the peristaltic wave progressing down the esophageal body. The intraluminal pressure recorded by the transducer is a function of the oncoming wave and the outflow resistance at the LES. If incomplete relaxation occurs, the resistance to outflow increases and the transducer records a higher ramp or intrabolus pressure. When the contraction wave reaches "C", the transducer records the contraction at that level. At "D" the wave has moved distally and the luminal pressure falls to baseline. The median amplitude of the ramp intrabolus pressure after a swallow of 5 mL water in 53 asymptomatic volunteers measured at four different levels was 11 mmHg (95th percentile) and the median duration was 14.2 s. There was no difference in amplitude or duration at different levels. The ramp pressure was significantly increased in patients with a HLES and following a Nissen fundoplication operation. Massey et al. (2) obtained concurrent esophageal videofluoroscopic and intraluminal manometric recordings in supine normal volunteers using different bolus volumes and viscosities and abdominal compression. Intrabolus pressure increased with bolus volume, viscosity, and abdominal compression.

2. A contraction bolus pressure which precedes the esophageal contraction response;
3. The contraction response.

Ramp intrabolus pressure is a waveform seen on esophageal manometry that precedes the peristaltic upstroke resulting from a swallow and may be an indicator of outflow obstruction.

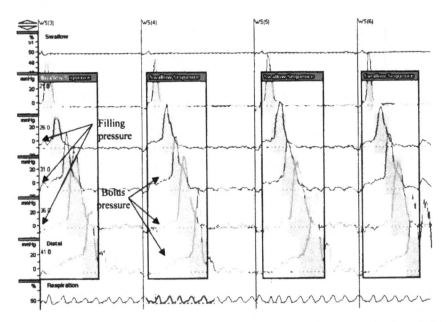

Figure 4.61 The filling and ramp intrabolus pressures are clearly seen in channels 3–6. Note that the duration of the ramp increases as the bolus distends the esophagus prior to esophageal contraction.

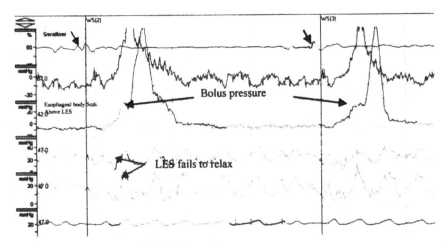

Figure 4.62 Increased intrabolus pressure is recorded in channel 2 which is 5 cm above the LES seen in channel 3. Note that the LES fails to relax in response to the swallow.

REFERENCES

1. Nisim AA, Bremner CG, Gastal OL, Johansson J, Campos GMR, Hashemi M, Lord RVN, Theisen J, Crookes PF, DeMeester TR. A manometric indicator of esophageal outflow resistance: ramp intrabolus pressure. Gastroenterology 1999; 116:50037 (abstr.).
2. Massey RJ, Dodds WJ, Kern MK, Brasseur JG, Shaker R, Harrington SS, Hogan WJ, Arndorfer RC. Determinants of intrabolus pressure during esophageal peristaltic bolus transport. Am J Physiol 1993; 264(3 Pt 1):G407–G413.

31. SCLERODERMA OF THE ESOPHAGUS [PROGRESSIVE SYSTEMIC SCLEROSIS (PSS)]

Description

Scleroderma of the esophagus describes the esophageal manifestations which occur in 75–85% of all patients with diffuse systemic sclerosis.

The esophageal abnormalities may predate the diagnosis of generalized scleroderma. The disease process affects only the smooth muscle of the esophagus, so that the upper striated muscle of the esophagus and the cricopharyngeal sphincter are normal. Scleroderma of the esophagus is characterized by a poor LES and hypomotility in the body of the esophagus (1).

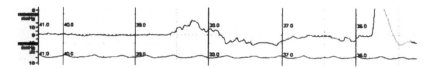

Figure 4.63   (Top) A short LES with a poor pressure. The patient has "scleroderma" of the esophagus.

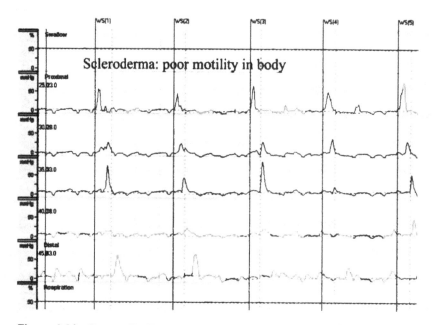

Figure 4.64   (Bottom) Swallow responses in the same patient are peristaltic but have very low pressures.

Motility features

- LES: low pressures at resting, poor swallow responses, normal coordination
- Body of Esophagus: hypomotile
- Cricopharyngeal sphincter: normal

Note: The manometric features are the same as that for IEM.

REFERENCE

1. Clements P, Kadell B, Ippoliti A, Ross M. Esophageal motility in progressive systemic sclerosis (PSS). Comparison of cine-radiographic and manometric evaluation. Dig Dis Sci 1979; 24:639–644.

32. MIXED CONNECTIVE TISSUE DISEASE

Description

A collagen-vascular disease which has clinical features found in progressive systemic sclerosis, polymyositis, and systemic lupus erythematosis (SLE), and is associated with high titers of a specific antibody from nuclear ribonuclarprotein antigen. More than 60% of these patients have esophageal involvement.

Motility features

Similar to those seen in PSS but are not usually as severe. The upper third of the esophagus may also be involved.

33. POLYMYOSITIS AND DERMATOMYOSITIS

Description

Diffuse inflammatory diseases of striated muscle and skin (dermatomyositis). Esophageal involvement occurs in 60–70% of patients.

Motility features

Decreased LES pressure in most patients. Decreased amplitude of esophageal peristalsis similar to the previous recording of scleroderma. Decreased UES pressure in many. Decreased amplitude of pharyngeal contractions in many (1,2).

REFERENCES

1. Jacob H, Berkowitz H, McDonald E, Beneventano T. The esophageal motility disorders of polymyositis. Arch Int Med 1988; 143:2262–2264.
2. Flick J, Boyle JT, Tuchman DN et al. Esophageal motor abnormalities in children and adolescents with mixed connective tissue disease. Pediatrics 1988; 82:107–111.

34. INEFFECTIVE ESOPHAGEAL MOTILITY (IEM)

Definition

A distinct manometric entity characterized by a hypocontractile esophagus in which the distal esophageal amplitudes are <30 mmHg or the contractions are nontransmitted in >30% of the wet swallows.

This is a reproducible manometric finding and is often associated with gastro-esophageal reflux. Leite et al. found that recumbent acid exposure in IEM did not differ significantly from that in patients with systemic sclerosis. They proposed that IEM should replace the term "nonspecific motility disorders" (NEMD) because 98% of NEMD patients have low or nontransmitted esophageal contractions. Kahrilas et al. noted peristaltic dysfunction with increasing severity in patients with esophagitis and, in a classic study by concurrent videofluroscopic and manometric recordings, showed that the mean peristaltic amplitude associated with instances of barium escape proximal to the peristaltic upstroke was 25 mmHg in the distal esophagus. (i.e., the minimal pressure amplitude required for regional volume clearance in supine subjects). The studies by Leite et al. (1) and Kahrilas et al. (2,3) are complementary and support the concept of inappropriate esophageal motility.

Note: An antireflux procedure "tailored" to the manometric features of the esophageal body responses has been popular in some centers, but has become controversial. Fibbe et al. randomized 200 patients into a "partial" (Toupet) fundoplication and a 360° fundoplication irrespective of the esophageal motility findings. Patients with dysmotility (>40% of contractions <20 mmHg pressure in the distal esophagus) had more severe esophagitis and a decreased LES pressure. The clinical outcome of both groups was similar at 4 months. A longer follow-up is clearly necessary to exclude a failing esophageal motility related to an imbalance of sphincter pressure and body capability.

Note: The surgeon should be very cautious if the global amplitude of the esophageal body contractions to wet swallows is <25 mmHg and if there are <25% effective contractions.

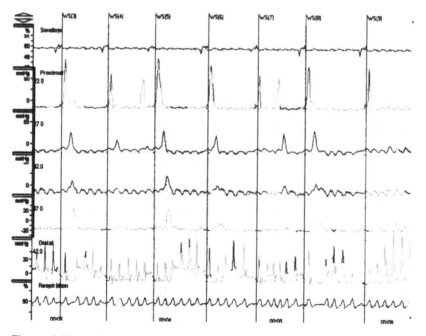

Figure 4.65 IEM. A wet swallow recording in the esophageal body. Four channels are in the esophageal body and the last channel is in the LES. The pressure responses in channels 2, 3, and 4 are very poor and are nontransmitted after some swallows.

REFERENCES

1. Leite LP, Johnston BT, Barrett J, Castell JA, Castell DO. Ineffective esophageal motility (IEM). The primary finding in pateints with nonspecific esophageal motor disorder. Dig Dis Sci 1997; 42:1859–1865.
2. Kahrilas PJ, Dodds WJ, Hogan WJ, Kern M, Arndorfer RC, Reece A. Esophageal peristaltic dysfunction in peptic esophagitis. Gastroenterology 1986; 92:897–904.
3. Kahrilis PJ, Dodds WJ, Hogan WJ. Effect of peristaltic dysfunction on esophageal volume clearance. Gastroenterology 1988; 94:73–78.

35. NONSPECIFIC ESOPHAGEAL MOTOR DISORDER (NSEMD)

Definition

An esophageal motility disorder which does not have features of a named motility disorder. Many of the features of NSEMD described in older classifications have been incorporated into the category of ineffective esophageal motility. However, there are still some unnamed features which are encountered and are included as NSEMD.

Manometric criteria (any of the following)

1. LES: Unexplained incomplete relaxation (residual pressure >7.5 mmHg).
2. Body: Simultaneous contractions not due to achalasia; Triple-peaked contractions; Retrograde contractions; Prolonged duration of contractions (mean >6 s), which are not diagnosed as DES.

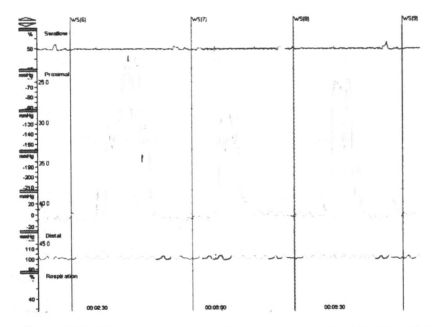

Figure 4.66 Triple-peaked contractions in response to a swallow. Double peaked responses are within the normal pattern of motility, but triple peaks do not occur in normal volunteers. The significance of this abnormality is unexplained but could be a harbinger of a more serious motility disorder.

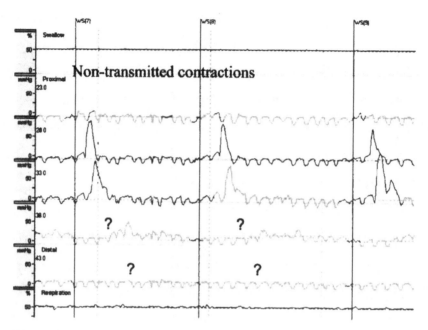

Figure 4.67 The swallow responses are not transmitted to the lower esophagus. This motility abnormality is unexplained.

36. CRICOPHARYNGEAL SPHINCTER

36.1. Background

The cricopharyngeal muscle is the major component of the UES. It is composed of striated muscle with predominantly slow twitch (Type 1) fibers, and has an abundance of fibroelastic connective tissue allowing it to expand to accommodate a 20-fold increase in flow rate with only a minimal increase in resistance (compliance).

Fibrosis of the UES, generally associated with aging, may impair the sphincters ability to open fully, thus causing an outflow resistance.

The relationship between UES compliance and the propulsive forces generated by the pharynx to achieve transsphincteric flow during a swallow has been masterly described using combined manometry and fluoroscopic imaging by Cook et al.

The swallow commences with the tongue pushing up against the hard palate, which imparts a piston-like force to the bolus. This propels the bolus into the pharynx at velocities of 40–50 cm/s. In the pharynx, the high-speed bolus slams up against the pharyngeal wall, and is driven around the epiglottis and downward into the mid pharynx. The UES opens just before the bolus arrives. Air precedes the bolus into the open UES. As the bolus flows through the UES it begins to slow down as frictional forces begin to plan an increasing dominant role. The flow rate through the sphincter is about 30–60 cm/s. Pressure and inertia are still dominant but friction assumes greater importance. As the bolus moves from the UES into the esophagus, it rapidly decelerates and slows to 2–4 cm/s. The stripping wave transforms into a peristaltic wave as rapid change gives way to slow change. Inertia gives way to friction. Thus, the dynamics of bolus flow in the upper esophageal segment is completely different to the characteristics in the lower esophagus.

When a swallow is iniated the hyoid moves superiorly and then anteriorly and elevates the larynx. At the same time the epiglottis closes. It has been observed that a drop to subatmospheric pressure is seen in approximately one-third of the subjects during a swallow. Brasseur et al. have shown that this drop corresponds closely to the instant at which the anterior–posterior walls of the UES separate and opening begins. At the time of UES opening the sudden anterior motion of the cricoid cartilage by anterior traction forces cause a momentary drop to subatmospheric pressure over a segment of about 2 cm in length. The subatmospheric pressure drop provides a nonradiological marker of UES opening.

36.2. Proximal PES Assessment

Before a swallow, the pressure transducers reflect atmospheric pressure. After the swallow is completed the pressure transducer will continue to read atmospheric pressure. The onset of the rise starts when any pressure movement >2 mmHg above the atmospheric baseline takes place. For dry swallows this will be the onset of the pharyngeal contraction (stripping) wave. For wet swallows this has been shown to reflect the head of the bolus entering this segment and subsequently reflects the hydrodynamic pressure within the bolus. A second upward slope occurs after ~0.35 s and represents the bolus tail and the subsequent closing pressure of the pharyngeal wall on the pressure transducer. *Therefore it is important to compare the tracing profile of the dry swallow with the wet swallows.* By performing this comparison it will be easy to distinguish the bolus pressure. This is important because often movement of the PES on the catheter, or the base of the tongue abutting against the catheter, will often cause a sharp upward rise in pressure. This can easily be confused with the bolus pressure but can be distinguished from it because it is also seen in the dry swallow.

The peak pharyngeal pressure can be measured as the highest amplitude attained during this event. An assessment of the pharyngeal stripping or clearing wave can be obtained by the time interval between successive peak pharyngeal pressures in the different channels of the manometric tracing.

The total duration of the pharyngeal event can therefore be measured. There is an association between radiological pooling and a prolonged pharyngeal interval.

36.3. Distal PES Including the Cricopharyngeal Muscle

Before the swallow the pressure profile in the UES will be elevated above the atmospheric baseline and equivalent to the resting UES pressure.

In the more proximal segment of the UES there may be a rise in the actual pressure before a fall is seen. Although the rise may actually represent the onset of the swallow, for assessment purposes we use the pressure drop. The lowest pressure reached in this segment is termed the minimal residual (MinR) pressure. The time taken for the minimal residual pressure to be reached relative to the onset is of crucial importance. *Normally this occurs just before or very close to the onse of the swallow.* The pressure is very often subatmospheric and will therefore have a negative value. This indicates sphincter opening. The next pressure measured is the maximal residual (MaxR) pressure. This is the pressure obtained after the Min residual pressure. It coincides with the bolus pressure seen on the more proximal channels in the pharynx. It always occurs after the onset of the swallow and represents the actual pressure caused by the bolus as it passes through the sphincter. The next point of interest is the pressure and time taken just before lumen closure in the UES when there is again an abrupt rise in pressure.

This is the contraction pressure and represents closure of the eosphageal lumen against the catheter sidehole and occurs just after the bolus tail leaves this segment. The final point of interest is the maximum pressure reached.

36.4. Outflow Resistance and "Compliance"

An evaluation of the outflow resistance and compliance is achieved by measuring the increase in bolus pressure to increasing volumes of swallowed bolus. This is the hydro-dynamic pressure within the bolus as it flows through the sphincter.

36.4.1. Normal Features of Cricopharyngeal Sphincter Manometry

The features listed below are normal. Any deviation from these features will indicate both an abnormality and the nature of the problem.

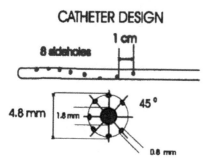

Figure 4.68 The 8-holed catheter used for the detailed cricopharyngeal sphincter study. The cri-copharyngeal sphincter mechanism can be measured using solid-state, Dent sleeve, or perfusion techniques. Because of the narrow width of the UES 91 cm) a spacing of at least 1 cm between manometric ports is necessary to capture the spatial pressure of the UES, and this is best achieved with microperfusion manometry which records an extremely high spatial resolution (18) Solid-state manometry has the disadvantage of high cost and transducer spacing.

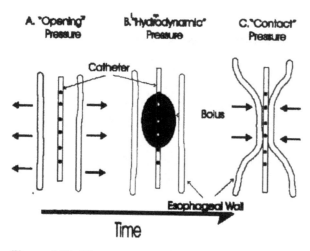

Figure 4.69 Three pressures acting on the recording catheter. The "opening" pressure is due to a mechanical muscle contraction force which pulls the cricopharyngeal muscle open. The bolus pushes against the muscle and when it has passed the cricopharyngeal muscle resumes its contracted state.

- The Bolus pressure does not increase significantly with increasing bolus volumes.
- The pharyngeal stripping wave shows progression from the more proximal channel to distal.
- The MinR pressure occurs before or approximately at the onset of the swallow.

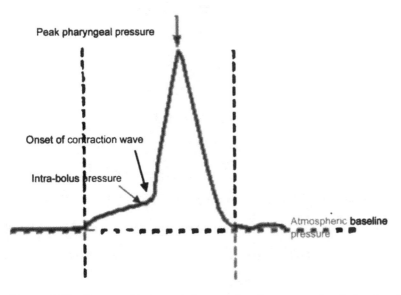

Figure 4.70   Pharyngeal bolus and pharyngeal peak pressures. A catheter placed in the pharynx will record a bolus pressure followed by a contraction wave.

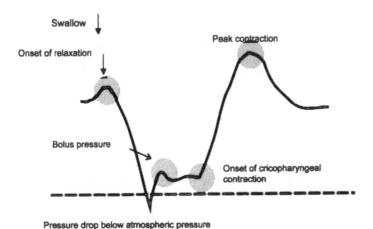

Figure 4.71   Cricopharyngeal pressure pattern. A catheter placed in the cricopharyngeal segment will record the events of a swallow. Note that the pressure has dropped below atmospheric pressure. This occurs in about one-third of swallows. The pressure above the baseline or minimal residual pressure, is 2.3–3.2 (see Table 36.6). This is followed by a short pressure rise (bolus pressure), before the cricopharyngeal contraction takes place. If the pressure does not fall below baseline, an opening problem is suspected. The pressure above the baseline is termed the "minimal residual pressure."

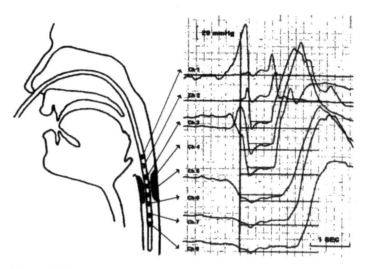

Figure 4.72 The complete recording using the 8-port catheter. Channels 1–2 are recording in the pharynx, 3–5 are in the cricopharyngeus muscle position and 6–8 are in the esophagus.

- The MinR pressure is lower than the Max Residual and always precedes the MaxR pressure.
- The Minimum residual pressure is often subatmospheric.

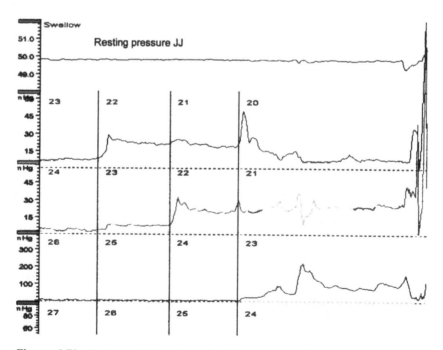

Figure 4.73 Resting pull-through study of the upper esophageal (cricopharyngeal) sphincter. The patient was asked not to swallow while the catheter was pulled through the sphincter. Three recordings of resting pressure were made.

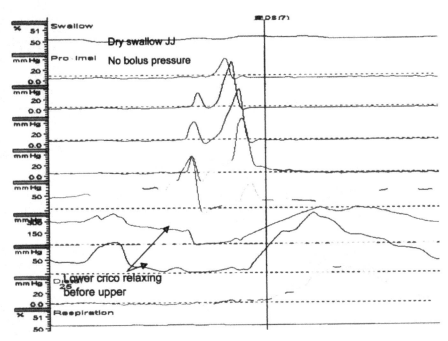

Figure 4.74 Normal relaxation of the UES. Wet swallow. 8-channel recording of a normal dry swallow. The upper 3 channels are in the pharynx and the lower 4–7 channels are in the sphincter. Channel 8 is in the upper esophagus. With a dry swallow a bolus pressure is not usually recorded. Note how the lower end of the sphincter relaxes first. The lowest point of relaxation (minimum residual pressure) is below the baseline atmospheric pressure, indicating normal relaxation. The upper limit of normal is 7 mm. Note that the sphincter pressure drop occurs at the onset of the bolus pressure recording.

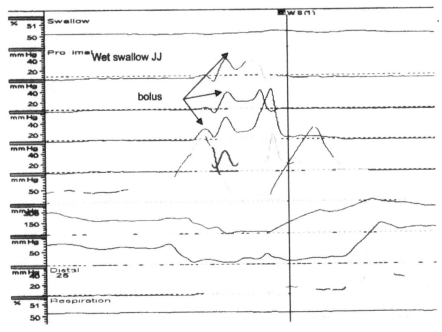

Figure 4.75 Normal relaxation of the UES. Wet swallow. A bolus pressure is noted during a wet swallow. Relaxation starts in the lower sphincter.

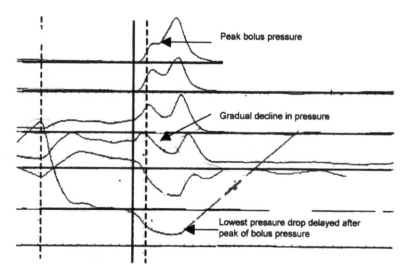

Figure 4.76 Features consistent with a relaxation problem. The pressure drop after a swallow occurs simultaneously in all the channels which measure UES pressure. The timing of the lowest pressure drop (Min residual pressure) is delayed and occurs after the pharyngeal bolus pressure (*instead of occurring at the onset of the bolus pressure rise*). If the bolus is the major contributor to the opening of the sphincter, then the pressure in the proximal channel will start to relax first followed by a gradual decline to the pressure equivalent to the pharyngeal bolus pressure. The min residual pressure in the proximal channel occurs before the min residual in the distal channel which indicates that the bolus is the major contributor to opening.

DECREASED COMPLIANCE

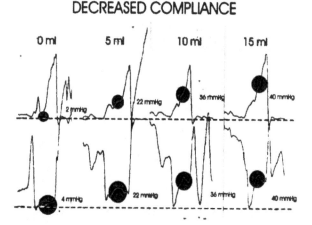

Figure 4.77 Feature indicating increased outflow resistance and a compliance problem. The pharyngeal bolus pressure increases with larger volumes of water. The increase is above normal values. Note the increase in bolus pressures with increases in bolus volumes from 0 to 15 mL water.

36.5. Effects of a Myotomy

A surgical myotomy will effectively abolish cricopharyngeal muscle tone. It will reduce the resting pressure and the pharyngeal contraction pressures. Therefore, it is indicated in patients who have poor UES relaxation. It does appear to improve sphincter opening. We have found a definite decrease in the MinR pressure postmyotomy. The timing also occurs earlier, and is most probably related to the improved hyolaryngeal excursion. Myotomy most probably has minimal effect on the intrinsic compliance of the pharyngeal musculature. However, the improved opening and relaxation results in a greater accommodation capacity of the pharynx and a decreased outflow resistance. These factors alone will result in a decrease in the intrabolus pressure which we use indirectly to determine muscle compliance.

36.6. Normal Values

Normal values obtained through SPT study are: length 5 cm (4.1–5.1), resting pressure 62.9 mmHg (41.3–87.2).

A detailed dynamic study is presented in the following table.

	Median	5th percentile	95th percentile
Length of UES (cm)	5.0	4.1	5.1
Resting pressure (mmHg)	61.0	40.0	87.0
Bolus pressure (mmHg)	13.3	11.2	15.7
Pharyngeal pressure (mmHg)	52.0	46.4	56.5
Minimal residual pressure (mmHg)	0.5	−2.3	3.2
Maximal residual pressure (mmHg)	11.3	8.9	14.5
Relaxation time (s)	0.58	0.546	0.60
Time of initiation of relaxation (s)			
Upper UES	−0.10	0.19	−0.43
Lower UES	−0.28	−0.401	−0.19

36.7. Advantages of Closely Spaced Water-Perfused Technique

	Water-perfused	Solid-state
Distinction between opening and relaxation	Yes	Poor
Assessment of opening	Yes	No
Compliance	Yes	Yes
Robust	Yes	No
Cheap	Yes	No
Catheter positioning	Simple	Difficult

36.8. Disadvantages

May not truly reflect peak pharyngeal pressure. Stimulation by the perfusate may be occasionally troublesome to patients.

REFERENCES

Bonington A, Mahon M, Whitmore I. A histological and histochemical study of the cricopharyngeus muscle in man. J Anat 1988; 156:27–37.

Brasseur JG, Hsieh P, Kern MK, Shaker R. Mathematical models of UES opening and transphincteric flow. Gastroenterology 1996; (AGA Abstracts).

Cerenko D, McConnel F, Jackson R.Quantitative assessment of pharyngeal bolus driving forces. Otolaryngol Head Neck Surg 1989; 100:57–63.

Cook IJ. Cricopharyngeal function and dysfunction (see comments). Dysphagia 1993; 8:244–251.

Cook IJ. Investigative techniques in the assessment of oro-pharyngeal dysphagia. Dig Dis 1998; 16:125–133.

Cook IJ, Blumbergs P, Cash K, Jamieson GG, Shearman DJ. Structural abnormalities of the cricopharyngeus muscle in patients with pharyngeal.

Cook IJ, Dodds WJ, Dantas RO, Massey B, Kern MK, Lang IM, Brasseur JG, Hogan WJ. Opening mechanisms of the upper esophageal sphincter. Am J Physiol Gastrointest Liver Physiol 1989; 257:G748–G759 (Abstr).

Dantos RO, Cook IJ, Dodds WJ, Kern MK, Lang IM, Brasseur JG. Biomechanics of cricopharyngeal bars. Gastroenterology 1990; 99(5):1269–1274.

Ergun GA, Kahrilas PJ, Lin S, Logemann JA, Harig JM. Shape, volume, and content of the deglutitive pharyngeal chamber imaged by ultra fast computerized tomography. Gastroenterology 1993; 105:1396–1403.

Jacob P, Kahrilas PJ, Logemann JA, Shah V, Ha T. Upper esophageal sphincter opening and modulation during swallowing. Gastroenterology 1989; 97:1469–1478.

Kahrilas PJ, Dodds WJ, Dent J, Logemann JA, Shaker R. Upper esophageal sphincter function during deglutition. Gastroenterology 1988; 95:52–62.

Kahrilas PJ, Logemann JA, Krugler C, Flanagan E. Volitional augmentation of upper esophageal sphincter opening during swallowing. Am J Physiol 1991; 260:G450–G456.

Kahrilas PJ, Logemann JA, Lin S, Ergun GA. Pharyngeal clearance during swallowing: a combined manometric and videofluoroscopic study. Gastroenterology 1992; 103:128–136.

Kahrilas PJ, Lin S, Logemann JA, Ergun GA, Facchini F. Deglutitive tongue action: volume accommodation and bolus propulsion. Gastroenterology 1993; 104:152–162.

Kristmundsdottir F, Mahon M, Froes MM, Cumming WJ. Histomorphometric and histopathological study of the human cricopharyngeus muscle: in health and in motor neuron disease. Neuropathol Appl Neurobiol 1990; 16:461–475.

Mason RJ, Bremner, CG. Myotomy for pharyngeal swallowing disorders. Adv Surg 1999; 33:375–384.

Williams RB, Anupam P, Brasseur JG, Cook IJ. Space-time pressure structure of pharyngoesophageal segment during swallowing. Am J Physiol—Gastrointest Liver Physiol 2001; 281:G1290–G1300.

37. EVALUATION OF RECURRENT SYMPTOMS AFTER ANTIREFLUX SURGERY

Heartburn, dysphagia, regurgitation, epigastric pain, and gas-bloat may result or recur after antireflux surgery. Esophageal motility and pH testing may be of value in the assessment of the following symptoms:

1. Recurrent heartburn due to reflux from a disrupted fundoplication. A mechanically defective LES and a positive pH score are diagnostic.

2. Recurrent symptoms due to a recurrent hiatal hernia. A double hump and double respiratory reversals may be evident on motility.

3. Dysphagia due to a fundoplication which is too tight or too long. A LES pressure which exceeds the swallow response pressure in the lower esophagus, and which may be >5 cm long or fails to relax effectively, may be the cause of the symptoms. A bolus pressure >20 mmHg is suggestive of a tight Nissen fundoplication.

4. Dysphagia and reflux symptoms due to a "slipped" Nissen fundoplication. A manometric pressure profile may suggest that the position of the fundoplication is well below the hiatus and the LES.

5. Chest pain due to a hypercontracting esophagus may be secondary to outflow obstruction from a tight or twisted Nissen fundoplication. An increased bolus pressure is also suggestive of an outflow obstruction.

Note: A paraesophageal hernia may cause dysphagia and pain. This complication is best diagnosed on a videoesophagram.

After a Nissen fundoplication the mean residual pressure in the LES following a wet swallow increases to ~7 mmHg (SD 3.2 mmHg) pressure, as compared to normal volunteers (4.0 mmHg SD 2.4).

REFERENCES

Crookes PF, Ritter MP, Johnson MP, Bremner CG, Peters JH, DeMeester TR. Static and dynamic function of the lower esophageal sphincter before and after laparoscopic Nissen fundoplication. J Gastrointest Surg 1997; 1:499–504.

Fibbe C, Layer P, Keller J, Strate U, Emmerman A, Zornig C. Esophageal motility in reflux disease before and after fundoplication: a prospective randomized clinical and manometric study. Gastroenterology 2001; 121:5–14.

38. NISSEN FUNDOPLICATION TOO TIGHT

Case history

Following a Nissen fundoplication the patient complained of chest pain, heartburn, and increased belching.

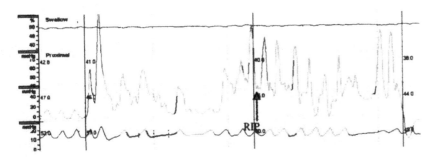

Figure 4.78 Motility study: The LES pressure was about 30 mmHg at the RIP (a HLES). The overall length of the LES was 3.6 cm and the abdominal length 1.6 cm (normal). Diagnosis: HLES.

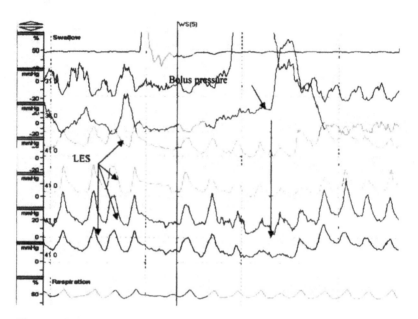

Figure 4.79 Relaxation study. The HLES relaxed incompletely. Channels 4–7 are in the sphincter area.

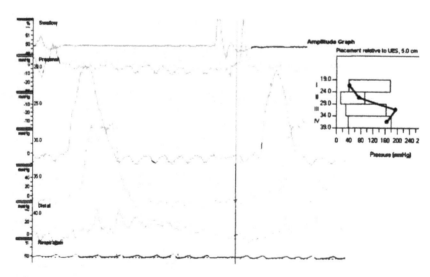

Figure 4.80 Swallow responses in the esophageal body were hypertensive. Inset: Graphic display of the body responses in segments I–IV.

A pH study confirmed that there was no increased acid exposure in the esophagus.

Assessment

The Nissen fundoplication was too tight and required revisional surgery.

39. POST NISSEN FUNDOPLICATION: RECURRENT HERNIA WITH INTACT FUNDOPLICATION

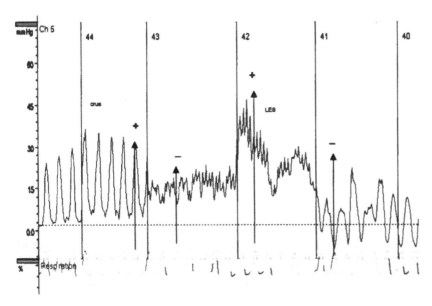

Figure 4.81 A double hump is present. The LES has separated from the crus. There is also a changing respiratory reversal from positive to negative and back to positive, a feature seen in motility recordings of some hiatal hernias.

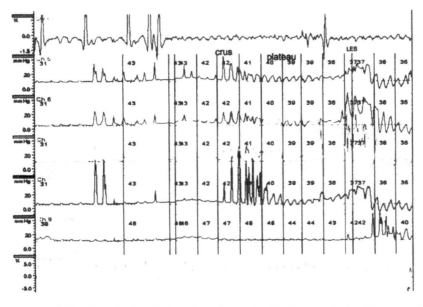

Figure 4.82 Motorized pull-through study of the LES in a patient with recurrent symptoms following a Nissen fundoplication operation. A double hump is seen in all four channels: the spacing between the humps suggests a 4 cm hernia.

40. POST NISSEN FUNDOPLICATION: NUTCRACKER ESOPHAGUS

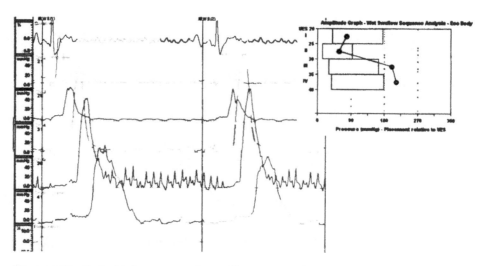

Figure 4.83 Peristaltic hypercontracting swallow responses in a patient who complained of chest pain and dysphagia following a Nissen fundoplication. Inset: graphic display of the swallow responses which are in the nutcracker range in segments III and IV.

REFERENCE

Fibbe C, Layer P, Keller J, Strate U, Emmerman A, Zornig C. Esophageal motility in reflux disease before and after fundoplication: a prospective randomized clinical and manometric study. Gastroenterology 2001; 121:5–14.

41. UNUSUAL PATTERNS

41.1. Achalasia with Hiatal Hernia

A patient with existing hiatal hernia and gastroesophageal reflux may develop achalasia. The onset of achalasia may coincide with the cessation of heartburn and the onset of dysphagia.

Manometric features

1. Lower sphincter:
   Double hump with plateau.
   LES may be hypertensive.
   Nonrelaxation or poor relaxation of the LES.
2. Body:
   Pressurized esophagus.
   Absent peristalsis.
   Hypomotility (normal amplitude of contractions in vigorous achalasia).

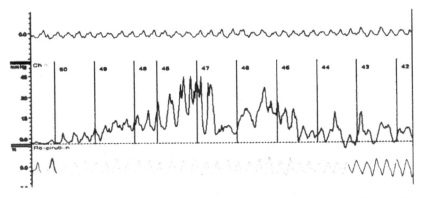

Figure 4.84   A SPT pressure profile in a patient who presented with a history of heartburn and increasing dysphagia. A double hump is clearly evident, and suggests a small hiatal hernia. The esophagus is pressurized.

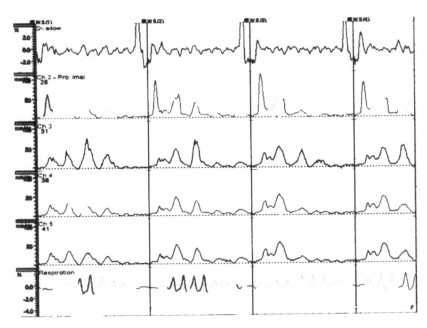

Figure 4.85   Swallow studies in the body of the esophagus show mirror image responses which are hypomotile.

41.2. HLES and Nutcracker Esophagus

Manometric features

1. LES:
    LES pressure greater than the 95th percentile of normal (26 mmHg).
    Normal relaxation of the lower sphincter.
2. Body:
    No pressurization. Body has a negative pressure relative to baseline intragastric pressure.
    Swallow responses > 180 mmHg.

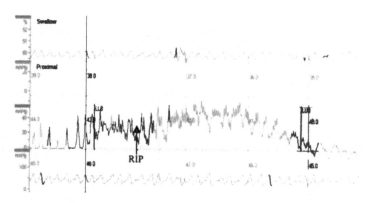

Figure 4.86 The LES is hypertensive on a SPT study (pressure 30 mmHg, normal range 6.1–25.6 mmHg). There is no evidence of pressurization in the esophageal body because the esophageal pressure is negative in the chest.

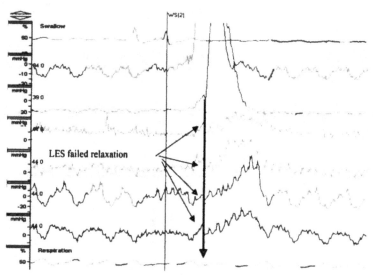

Figure 4.87 Relaxation study: four channels are at the same level within the lower esophageal sphincter. Swallow-induced relaxation failed.

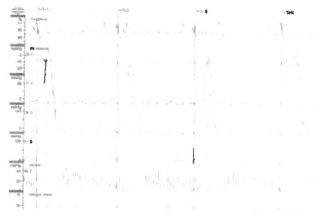

Figure 4.88 Swallow responses in the body show pressures >180 mmHg ("Nutcracker range").

41.3. Hiatal Hernia with a HLES

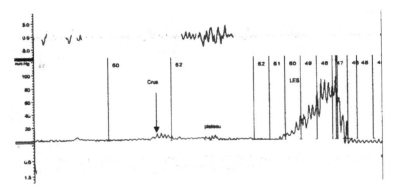

Figure 4.89 A compressed recording to include the double hump and plateau of a hiatal hernia. The lower sphincter pressure is hypertensive.

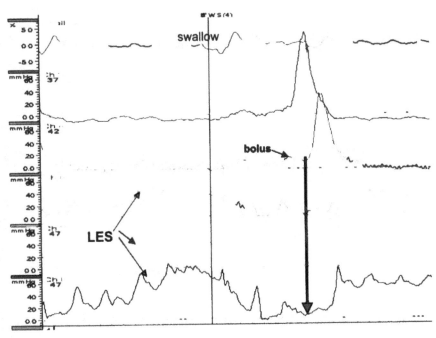

Figure 4.90 Relaxation study of the HLES. Relaxation is complete in this example but may be incomplete in this condition.

41.4. End-Stage GERD

Manometric features

1. Mechanically defective LES;
2. Hypomotility in esophageal body with loss of peristalsis.

Comment: Technically the features resemble a treated achalasia (disrupted LES, hypomotility, no peristalsis, absent pressurization). A defective LES and hypomotility pattern is also seen in scleroderma of the esophagus and in end-stage GERD.

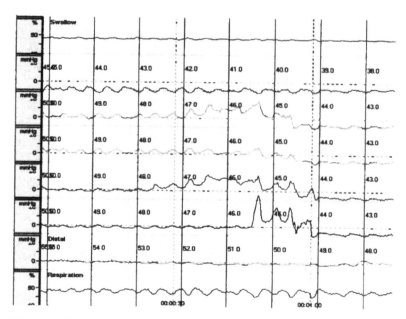

Figure 4.91 Motorized pull-through study on a grossly obese patient with severe GERD and regurgitation. The LES in all four channels has a low pressure.

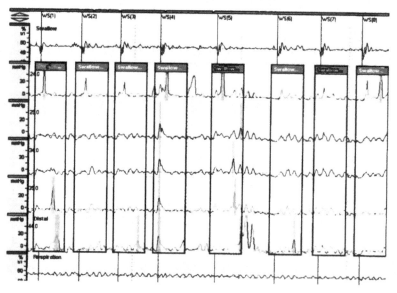

Figure 4.92 Poor responses to swallows which are hypomotile. There are also frequent simultaneous contractions (the features of those of IEM).

41.5. HLES with Pressurized Esophagus

Case history

A 76-year-old female patient complained of heartburn (30% relief with PPI therapy), dysphagia requiring multiple swallows to get food down, epigastric pain and excess mucus from the throat.

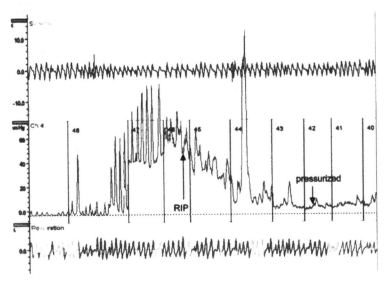

Figure 4.93 LES study showed a resting pressure which was hypertensive (mean pressure 50.4 mmHg). The body of the esophagus is pressurized.

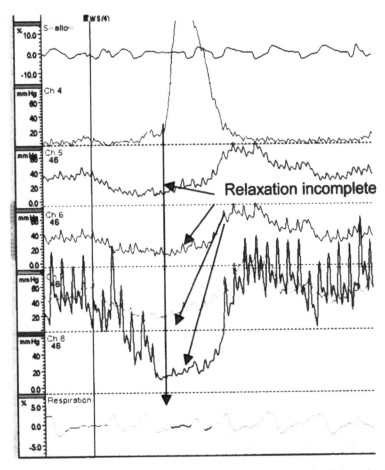

Figure 4.94 Relaxation study showed incomplete relaxation in all four channels.

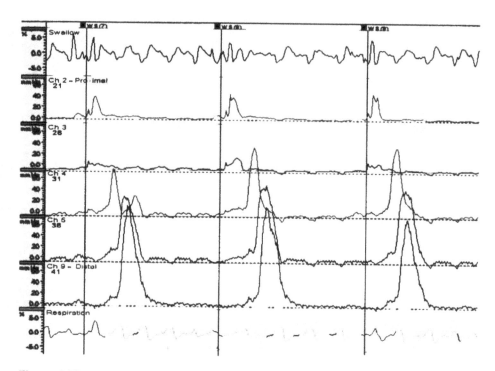

Figure 4.95 Body study showed normal peristalsis which excluded achalasia.

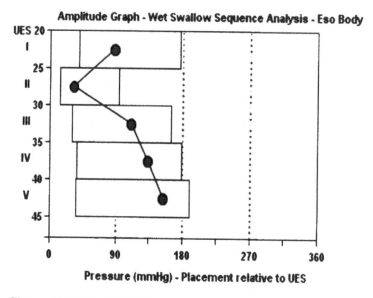

Figure 4.96 Graphic display of normal amplitude in Sections I–V. Each section represents a 5 cm segment of esophagus.

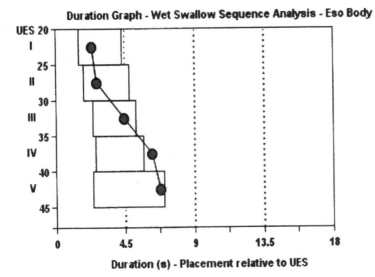

Figure 4.97 Graphic display of duration of swallow responses which was at the extreme upper end of the 95th percentile of normal.

The patient had a HLES which relaxed incompletely, and an elevated intrabolus pressure suggesting an outflow obstruction.

41.6. Epiphrenic Diverticulum (1)

An epiphrenic diverticulum is a pulsion diverticulum due to outflow obstruction at the LES. It may be associated with achalasia, a HLES or a nonrelaxing LES. A raised intra-bolus pressure and a nonrelaxing LES is highly suggestive of outflow obstruction.

Case history
A 48-year-old male patient complained of intermittent dysphagia for solids and liquids, frequent bouts of chest pain, occasional regurgitation and heartburn. A videoesophagram demonstrated an epiphrenic diverticulum.

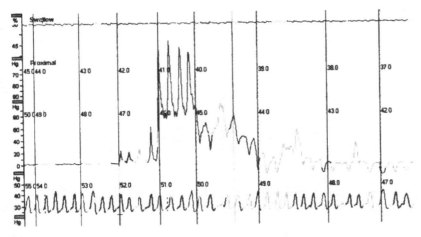

Figure 4.98 Manometric study demonstrated a HLES.

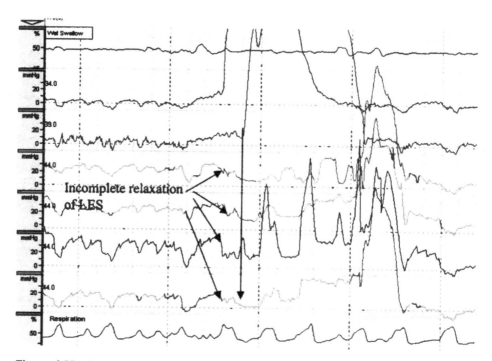

Figure 4.99 A swallow study showed incomplete relaxation of the LES.

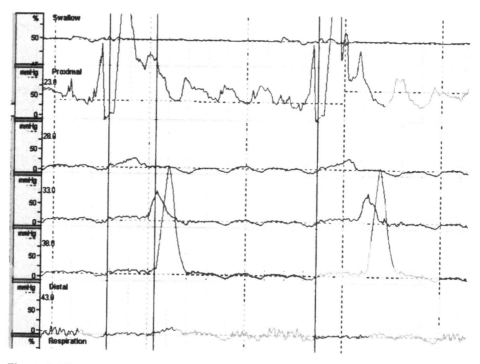

Figure 4.100 Body swallow study. The contractions in the lower esophagus were hypertensive (nutcracker range).

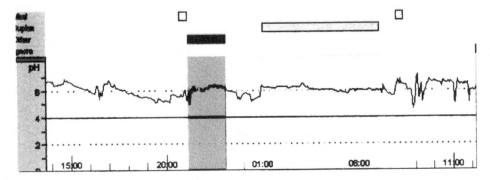

Figure 4.101 pH study. There was no acid exposure in the esophagus.

REFERENCE

1. Nehra D, Lord RV, DeMeester TR, Theisen J, Peters JH, Crookes PF, Bremner CG. Physiologic basis for the treatment of epiphrenic diverticulum. Ann Surg 2002; 235(3):346–354.

42. AMBULATORY MOTILITY

Ambulatory motility overcomes some of the shortcomings of stationary manometry and, in particular, the brevity of the test which is performed in an unphysiological environment (starved patient studied in the supine position and with liquid swallows only). Only 10 swallows of liquid are analyzed in a stationary manometric study, whereas more than 1000 are computerized during ambulatory motility study and with swallows of both liquid and solid food. Mathematically, the chances of detecting an abnormal contraction which occurs 10% of the time is only 0.65 if a stationary study is performed. The probability of detecting this same abnormality by ambulatory manometry is almost a certainty. The incorporation of pH analysis with ambulatory manometry data allows an assessment of esophageal clearance of refuxed acid as well as the ability to identify the effects of esophageal acidification or esophageal motility.

Included in this section are results of normal values, esophageal function in gastroesophageal reflux disease, achalasia, hypertensive lower esophageal sphincter, diffuse esophageal spasm, non-specific esophageal motor disorders, and Barrett's esophagus.

The software for this analysis was supplied by Medtronic. The validation of the analysis was described in a Ph.D. dissertation (Bremner RM. Ambulatory Motility. Ph.D. dissertation, University of Witwatersrand, 1995).

42.1. Normal Patterns

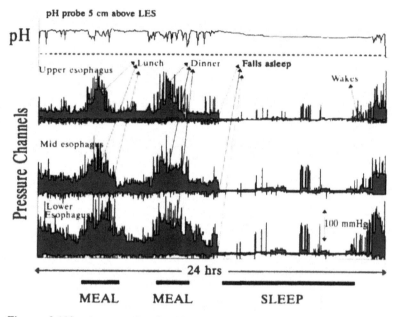

Figure 4.102 An example of a 24 h pH and manometry recording in the compressed mode showing the full 24 h of study.

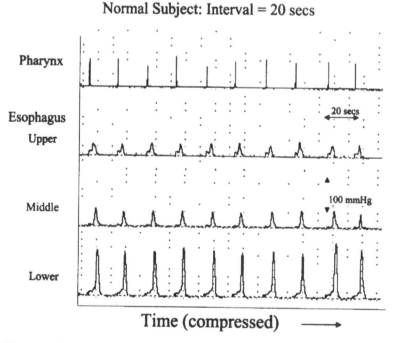

Figure 4.103 An example of the recording of esophageal pressures in a normal subject when the interval between swallows is 20 s.

Normal Subject: Interval = 5 secs

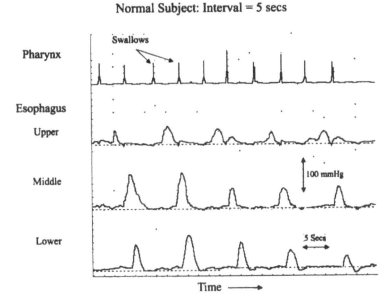

Figure 4.104 Example of a recording of esophageal pressures in a normal subject while eating a meal (recording taken at an interval of 5 s). Note the variation in the amplitudes of contractions.

42.2. Gastroesophageal Reflux Disease

Contraction amplitudes decrease with increasing severity of acid reflux injury. The ability to increase the amplitude of contractions in the lower esophagus during mealtimes is compromised, although similar amplitudes of contractions in the interprandial periods may be the same as in normals (Table 4.6).

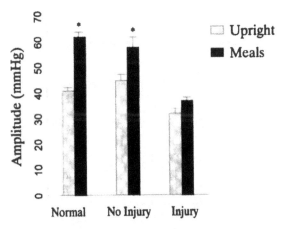

Figure 4.105 Mean amplitude of contractions for the upright and meal periods in normal subjects and patients with gastroesophageal reflux disease. *$p < 0.05$ vs. upright.

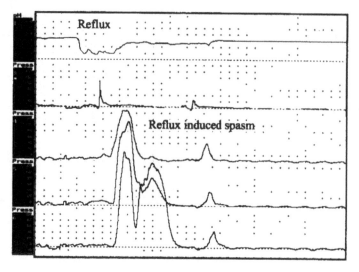

Figure 4.106   Example of a recording demonstrating the reflux-induced "spasm."

Table 4.6   Ambulatory Motility Characteristics of Normal Subjects and Patients with GERD

Parameter	Normals ($n = 25$)	No injury ($n = 26$)	Injury ($n = 19$)
Amplitude (mmHg)			
Upright			
Channel 1	34 ± 2	33 ± 2	31 ± 2
Channel 2	40 ± 2	40 ± 2	32 ± 3[a,b]
Channel 3	42 ± 2	45 ± 4	32 ± 2[a,b]
Meal			
Channel 1	47 ± 2	41 ± 3	41 ± 4
Channel 2	54 ± 3	51 ± 4	37 ± 4[a,b]
Channel 3	62 ± 4	58 ± 6	37 ± 3[a,b]
Supine			
Channel 1	35 ± 2	33 ± 2	27 ± 2
Channel 2	47 ± 3	47 ± 3	32 ± 3[a,b]
Channel 3	51 ± 3	54 ± 5	32 ± 3[a,b]
Multipeaked (%) (distal esophagus)			
Upright	0.4 ± 0.2	0.6 ± 0.1	0.7 ± 0.1[a]
Meal	0.7 ± 0.3	0.7 ± 0.3	2.2 ± 0.6[a,b]
Supine	1.7 ± 0.5	1.2 ± 0.3	1.9 ± 0.4
Peristaltic Waves (%)			
Upright	82 ± 2.3	75 ± 1.8	72 ± 2.8[a]
Meal	89 ± 1.0	84 ± 1.6	79 ± 2.7
Suprine	71 ± 2.6	59 ± 2.0	69 ± 3.3

(*continued*)

Table 4.6 *Continued*

Parameter	Normals ($n = 25$)	No injury ($n = 26$)	Injury ($n = 19$)
Effective (%)			
Upright	35 ± 3.2	30 ± 3.1	18 ± 2.8[a,b]
Meal	53 ± 2.6	41 ± 3.3	29 ± 4.3[a,b]
Suprine	31 ± 3.0	25 ± 2.4	15 ± 2.4[a,b]
Ineffective (%)			
Upright	40 ± 2.9	52 ± 2.7	60 ± 3.0[a,b]
Meal	30 ± 1.9	43 ± 2.4	52 ± 4.5[a,b]
Suprine	57 ± 3.0	68 ± 2.3	67 ± 3.2[a]

[a] $p < 0.01$ vs. normals.
[b] $p < 0.01$ vs. no injury.
Note: Channel 1, 2, and 3 are 15, 10, and 5 cm above the LES, respectively; Channel 3 = distal.

Motor abnormalities may result from reflux episodes. As the amplitude of contractions decreases, the prevalence of multipeaked pressure responses increases and the percentage of effective contractions decreases.

42.3. Hypertensive LES

Description

Esophageal body manometry may reveal an increased bolus pressure and esophageal spasm in patients who have a hypertensive lower esophageal sphincter (HTLES) on stationary motility studies. The increased bolus pressure is a measure of outflow resistance, and is manifest especially during mealtimes. An ambulatory diagnosis of diffuse esophageal spasm or nutcracker esophagus has been made in patients with stationary motility diagnosis of hypertensive lower esophageal sphincter. During mealtimes the amplitude and duration of contraction waves increases, and the percentage of peristaltic waves decreases (Table 4.7).

Table 4.7 Ambulatory Motility Characteristics of Normal Subjects and Patients with HTLES

Parameter	Normals	HTLES	Significance
Amplitude (mmHg)			
Upright			
Channel 1	35 ± 3	42 ± 5	NS
Channel 2	40 ± 2	58 ± 7	$p = 0.006$
Channel 3	43 ± 3	69 ± 6	$p = 0.001$
Meal			
Channel 1	49 ± 3	50 ± 4	NS
Channel 2	57 ± 4	71 ± 7	NS
Channel 3	68 ± 4	85 ± 8	$p = 0.039$

(continued)

Table 4.7 *Continued*

Parameter	Normals	HTLES	Significance
Supine			
Channel 1	40 ± 3	35 ± 3	NS
Channel 2	50 ± 3	61 ± 9	NS
Channel 3	53 ± 3	66 ± 7	NS
Duration (s)			
Meals			
Channel 1	2.41 ± 0.13	2.28 ± 0.17	NS
Channel 2	2.28 ± 0.15	2.71 ± 0.15	$p = 0.04$
Channel 3	2.38 ± 0.11	2.98 ± 0.21	$p = 0.01$
Peristaltic Waves (%)			
Upright	81 ± 2.7	60 ± 4.2	$p = 0.0002$
Meal	88 ± 1.4	78 ± 3.8	NS
Supine	68 ± 2.5	51 ± 5.3	$p = 0.015$
Efficacy (%)			
Upright	36 ± 4.0	30 ± 5.3	NS
Meal	56 ± 2.7	53 ± 6.3	NS
Supine	32 ± 3.2	15 ± 3.4	$p = 0.003$

42.4. Achalasia

Description

An increase in baseline pressure during meals is typical of untreated achalasia, and corresponds to the retention of food in the esophageal body (Fig. 4.109). This increase is minimal or absent in patients who have undergone myotomy.

A high prevalence of isobaric repetitive contractions during meals is frequently present, and these also decrease after myotomy (Fig. 4.110). Occasional peristalsis may be observed. Prolonged monitoring of the esophageal body and lower esophageal sphincter has been described using a multi-lumen assembly incorporating a Dent sleeve connected to a portable water perfused manometric system (1). Prolonged manometry in achalasia patients revealed the occurrence of complete LES relaxations, transient lower esophageal relaxations (TLESRs), variations in LES pressure associated with a meal or phase 111, and high amplitude and retrograde esophageal pressure waves.

REFERENCE

1. van Herwaarden MA, Samson M, Smout AJ. Prolonged manometric recordings of esophagus and lower esophageal sphincter in achalasia patients. Gut 2001; 49(6):813–821.

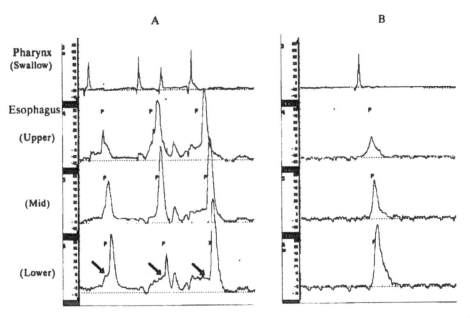

Figure 4.107 Example of the ambulatory recording of a patient with HLES during a meal (A) and during the interprandial period (B). Note the prominent intrabolus pressures in A (arrows).

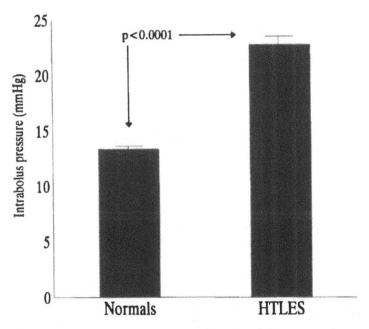

Figure 4.108 Mean ± standard error for the intrabolus pressures in normal subjects and patients with HLES.

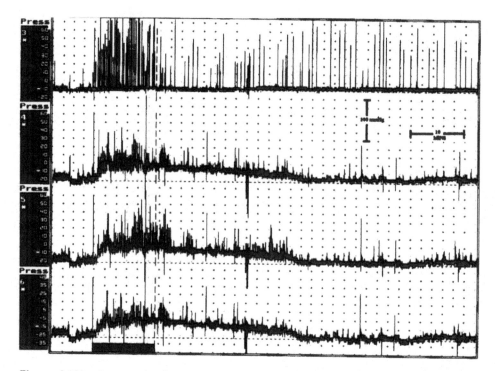

Figure 4.109 An example of a compressed record (80 min) showing an elevation in the baseline pressure that occurs with eating. The black bar in the bottom channel indicates the meal period.

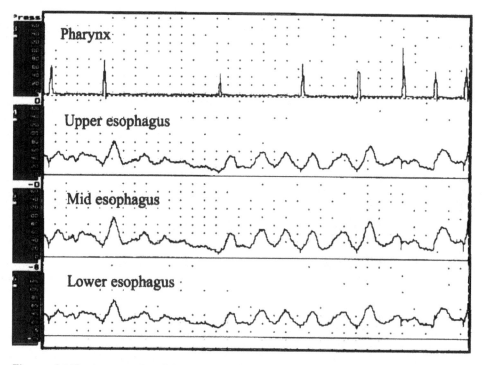

Figure 4.110 An example of the repetitive low amplitude isobaric contractions seen in the esophagus during meals. Note the elevation in baseline pressure. Time = 2 s between dots.

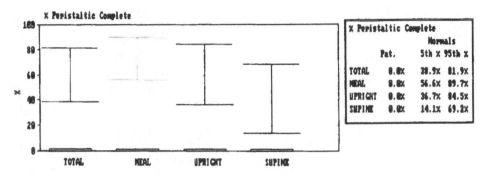

Figure 4.111 Computer analysis of the ambulatory motility recording in a patient with classic achalasia. Note the absence of complete peristaltic sequences.

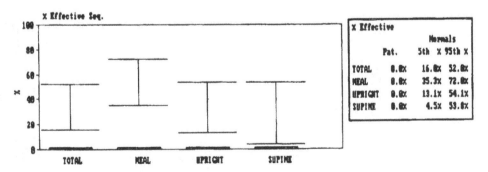

Figure 4.112 The same patient as above but the analysis reveals that partial peristalsis (in the upper esophagus) is present and that this increased during meals.

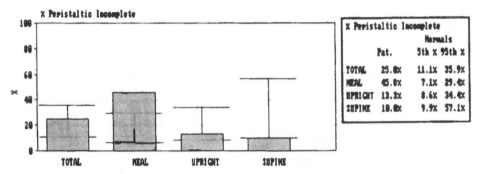

Figure 4.113 Although partial peristalsis can be present in the upper esophagus in patients with achalasia the absence of complete peristalsis translates to a propulsion failure that is, no effective peristaltic waves.

42.5. Diffuse Esophageal Spasm (DES)

Manometric features

Swallow responses have an increased amplitude, increased duration, and are multi-peaked; frequent simultaneous contractions during mealtimes; meal periods are also

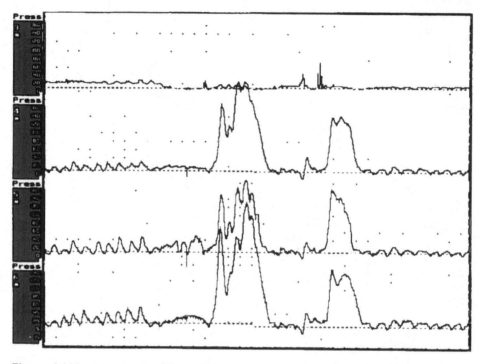

Figure 4.114 An example of the ambulatory recording of a patient with diffuse esophageal spasm, showing characteristic spastic contractions.

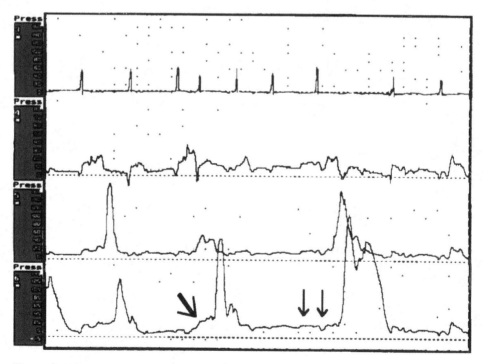

Figure 4.115 An example of increased bolus pressure in the lower esophagus on a patient with diffuse esophageal spasm. Note also the esophageal pressurization between swallows (↓).

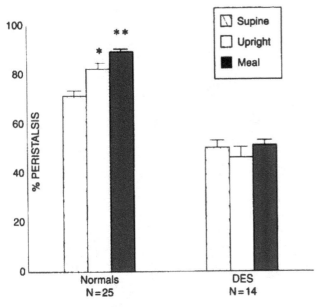

Figure 4.116 The prevalence of peristalsis during the different periods in normal subjects and DES patients. $^*p < 0.05$ vs. supine, $^{**}p < 0.05$ vs. upright.

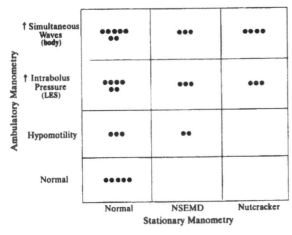

Figure 4.117 Classification of patients with non-obstructive dysphagia based on the functional defect. Ambulatory manometry may give a more precise classification of the motility disorder since the analysis is based on hundreds of contractions during both eating and interprandial periods.

characterized by repetitive simultaneous contractions which are not related to swallowing; frequent episodic high amplitude contractions of > 150 mmHg; High intrabolus pressures in the majority of swallow responses, indicating relative outflow obstruction; increased prevalence of multipeaked contractions; increased isolated contractions (not related to contractions in other levels) in the lower esophagus.

42.6. Cough

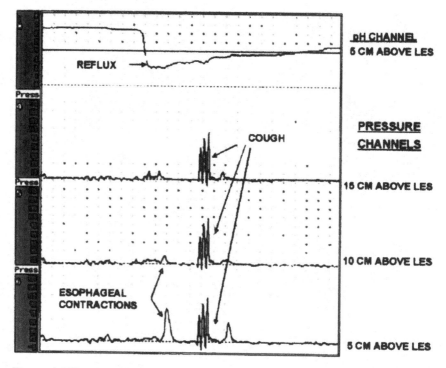

Figure 4.118 Reflux-induced coughing. The pH channel has recorded a reflux episode which is followed by coughing.

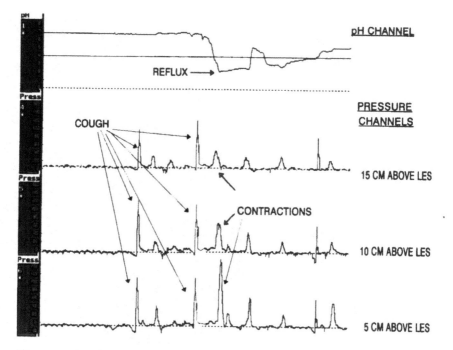

Figure 4.119 Cough-induced reflux. Coughing followed by a reflux episode.

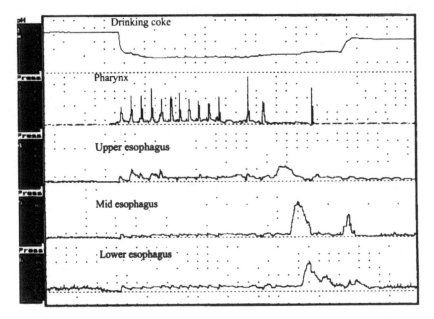

Figure 4.120 Spurious reflux: drinking beverages. The pH probe detects acidity in the esophagus. The pharyngeal probe records the frequent swallows when drinking. The upper and lower esophageal exhibit deglutitive inhibition, which is followed by a peristaltic wave resulting in clearing of the acidic beverage.

5
Ambulatory pH Monitoring

1. AMBULATORY pH MONITORING: HISTORICAL MILESTONES

1935   Winkelstein coined the term "peptic esophagitis," recognizing that reflux of acid gastric contents were responsible.

1958   Bernstein and Baker developed the acid perfusion test.

1960   Tuttle, Bettavello, and Grossman showed that heartburn coincided with a fall in pH below 4. They used probe to diagnose reflux.

1964   Miller described continuous pH monitoring for 12–24 h.

1961   Hill described pH measurement at the gastroesophageal junction.

1969   Spencer reported on prolonged pH monitoring in patients with gastro-esophageal reflux.

1970   Patrick and Woodward continued the use of pH monitoring in symptomatic patients.

1974   Johnson and DeMeester described the clinical use and quantitation of 24 h pH monitoring.

1980s   Small portable recorders were developed.

REFERENCES

Bernstein LM, Baker LA. A clinical test for esophagitits. Gastroenterology 1958; 34:760–781.

Hill LD, Morgan EH, Kellog HB. Experimentation as an aid in management of esophageal disorders. Am J Surg 1961; 102:240–252.

Johnson LF, DeMeester TR. Twenty-four hour pH monitoring of the distal esophagus: a quantitative measure of gastroesophageal reflux. Am J Gastroenterol 1974; 62:325–332.

Miller FA. Utilization of inlying pH probe for evaluation of acid-peptic diathesis. Arch Surg 1964; 89:199–203.

Patrick FG. Investigation of gastroesophageal reflux in various positions with a two-lumen pH probe. Gut 1970; 11:659–667.

Spencer J. Prolonged pH recording in the study of gastroesophageal reflux. Br J Surg 1969; 56:912–914.

Tuttle SG, Bettavello A, Grossman MI. Esophageal acid perfusion test and a gastroesophageal reflux test in patients with esophagitis. Gastroenterology 1960; 38:861–872.

Winkelstein A. Peptic esophagitis (a new clinical entity). J Am Med Assoc 1935; 104:906.

Woodward DAK. Response of the gullet to gastric reflux in patients with hiatal hernia and oesphagitis. Thorax 1970; 24:459–464.

2. EQUIPMENT

2.1. Electrodes

1. Glass electrodes are 1–3 mm in diameter, and are expensive but give the most accurate recordings (1). These are used for about 20 patients.
2. Antimony electrodes are 1.5 mm in diameter, more durable and cheaper. These are less reproducible and can be used on fewer patients.
3. ISFET pH electrodes (ion-sensitive field effect-transistor) have responses similar to glass electrodes and are smaller and cheaper.

2.2. Recording Systems

There are several manufacturers of compact portable recorders, which weigh between 150 and 397 g. They have similar sampling rates between 1 and 20 s, and memory sizes between 96 and 256 kB. All are equipped with event markers and are battery-driven. (Medtronic; Oakfield instruments; Medical Measurement Systems; Medical Instruments Corporation; Albyn Medical; Sandhill Scientific.)

2.3. Calibration

Details of calibration and performance of the study are given by the manufacturers and are available in specific texts.

3. PATIENT INSTRUCTIONS

Proton pump inhibitors are discontinued for 2 weeks, Cimetidine for 1 week, and antacids for 1 day. Dietary restrictions must be adhered to. Patients are instructed to push the event markers when they have meals and when they lie down (supine periods).

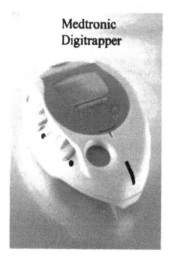
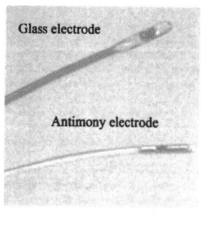

Figure 5.1   "Digitrapper" and pH probes used for ambulatory pH testing.

3.1. pH Test Diet

Patients may choose to eat any of the foods listed below during the 24 h test period.

Meat/Fish/Cheese	Grilled cheese sandwich, Macaroni and cheese, Cheese (American suggested), Roast beef (may have gravy, also beef), Salmon, Tuna, Tuna/noodle casserole, Chicken
Fruit	Bananas, Apples, Watermelon, Cantaloupe, Strawberries, Honeydew melon
Vegetables	Beans, Cabbage, Carrots, Corn, Peas, Potato (baked, mashed, fried, hashbrowns), Spinach, Sweet potatoes, Turnips
Beverages	Milk, Water, Tea, Coffee, No carbonated beverages, alcohol, or fruit juices
Other	Bread, Toast, Butter or margarine, Cream of chicken soup, Cream of mushroom soup, Chicken soups, Cream of wheat, Cereal, Eggs, Vanilla ice cream

4. SCORING SYSTEMS

The first and most widely used system is the DeMeester score which was quantified by Johnson and DeMeester in 1974.

Other systems used are the Kay (2) (postprandial), Branicki (3) (frequency-duration), and Vitale (4) (cumulative pH) systems.

The normal values derived from 50 healthy volunteers are listed in Table 5.1. The composite score is derived from six components of the analysis.

The Synectics System uses a Gastrosoft software program, which calculates the values and computes the final score. A DeMeester score >14.7 denotes an abnormally high acid exposure to the esophagus (5,6).

Table 5.1 Esophageal Acid Exposure in 50 Healthy Volunteers

	Mean	SD	Median	Minimum	Maximum	95%
Total time at pH less than 4 (%)	1.5	1.4	1.2	0	6.0	4.5
Upright time at pH less than 4 (%)	2.2	2.3	1.6	0	9.3	8.4
Supine time at pH less than 4 (%)	0.6	1.0	0.1	0	4.0	3.5
Number of episodes	19.0	12.8	16.0	2.0	56.0	46.9
Number of episodes ≥5 min	0.8	1.2	0	0	5.0	3.5
Longest episode (min)	6.7	7.9	4.0	0	46.0	19.8
Composite score	6.0	4.4	5.0	0.4	18.0	14.7

Note: SD, Standard deviation.

REFERENCES

1. DeMeester TR, Johnson LF, Joseph GJ et al. Pattern of gastroesophageal reflux in health and disease. Ann Surg 1976; 184:459–470.

2. Kay MD. Postprandial gastro-oesophageal reflux in healthy people. Gut 1977; 18:709–712.
3. Branicki FJ, Evans DJ, Joes JA et al. A frequency-duration index (FDI) for evaluation of ambulatory recording of gastro-oesophageal reflux. Br J Surg 1984; 71:425.
4. Vitale GC, Cheadle WG, Patel B et al. The effect of alcohol on nocturnal gastroesophgeal reflux. J Am Med Assoc 1987; 285:2077.
5. Bremner RM, Bremner CG, DeMeester TR. Gastroesophageal reflux: the use of pH monitoring. Curr Probl Surg 1995; 6:429–568.
6. Buckton GK, Evans DF, eds. Clinical Measurement in Gastroenterology. Vol 1. The Oesophagus. Oxford, UK: Blackwell Science, 1997.

4.1. Patterns of Esophageal Acid Exposure to the Esophagus

In normal asymptomatic people there is a small amount of acid exposure to the esophagus. Abnormal exposure may take place in the erect position, in the supine position, or in both positions. There may also be abnormal exposure in the postprandial period due to shortening of the lower esophageal sphincter when the stomach distends.

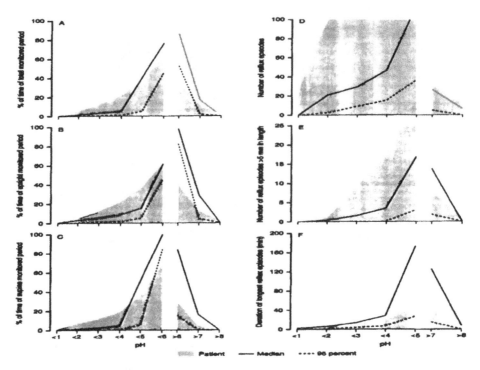

Figure 5.2 Graphic display of the six components of esophageal pH exposure showing the median and 95th percentile levels in 50 normal individuals with whole pH values above and below 6.0 as thresholds. The black area represents measurements made in a patient. When the black area exceeds the 95th percentile line for a given pH threshold, the patient is considered to have an abnormal value for the component measured. (A) Percent cumulative exposure for total time; (B) percent cumulative exposure for upright time; (C) percent cumulative exposure for supine time; (D) number of episodes; (E) number of episodes lasting longer than 5 min; and (F) length of longest reflux episode. (From Streets CG, DeMeester TR. Ambulatory 24 h esophageal pH monitoring. Why, when and what to do. J Clin Gastroenterol 2003; 37(1):14–22.)

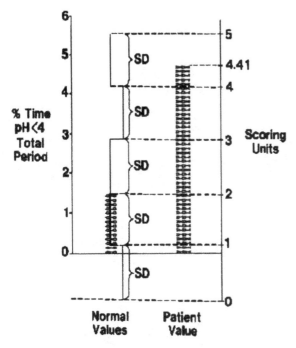

Figure 5.3 Concept of using the standard deviation as the scoring unit to score the component percent time when the pH was less than 4 for the total period. Note the establishment of an abstract 0.2 standard deviations below the mean value for total-period acid exposure measured in normal individuals. Theoretically, this allows scoring the measurement in patients as though the normal values were parametric.

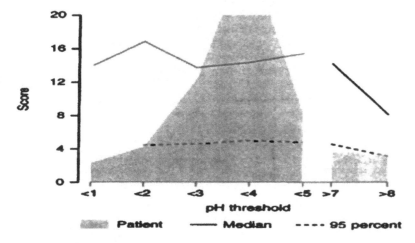

Figure 5.4 Graphic display of the composite score used to express the overall result of a 24 h esophageal pH recording. The lower line represents the median score and the upper line the 95th percentile of 50 normal subjects. The black area represents the composite score of the patient, with increased esophageal acid exposure measured at pH less than 4.

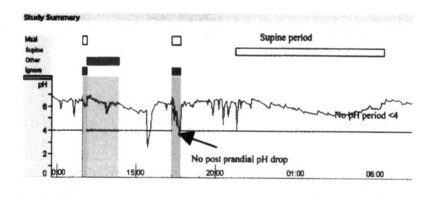

Figure 5.5   Recording of ambulatory pH monitoring in a normal patient. An analysis of the reflux events is shown in the table. The analysis confirms that there was no increase in acid exposure in the esophagus.

4.2. Use of a Double pH Probe

When there are suspected extra-esophageal reflux symptoms such as unexplained asthma, chronic cough, voice changes, recurrent laryngitis, or dental erosions, a double pH probe recording may assist in explaining the symptoms. The lower probe is placed in the usual position 5 cm above the upper border of the lower esophageal sphincter, and the upper probe is placed in the upper esophagus. Our standard position is 15 cm above the lower probe.

5. POSTPRANDIAL GASTROESOPHAGEAL REFLUX

A structurally intact and competent lower esophageal sphincter may shorten and become incompetent during gastric distention.

The 2 h postprandial acid exposure and lower esophageal sphincter characteristics in normal subjects ($n = 94$) is as follows.

	Mean	Median	SD	95th percentile
% Time at pH less than 4 in postprandial period	2.26	2.69	1.20	8.43
Number of pH less than 4 episodes in postprandial period	3.58	3.83	2.0	11.12
Time at pH less than 4 in postprandial period (min)	2.77	3.39	1.55	10.13
Number of episodes >5 min	0.22	0.59	0	2.0
Longest episode (min)	3.06	5.64	1.3	10.5
Total sphincter length (cm)	3.47	0.80	3.6	4.91
Intra-abdominal length (cm)	1.89	0.68	1.9	3.2
Sphincter pressure (mmHg)	15.02	6.14	13.15	26.2

Note: The postprandial time increases in patients with a defective lower esophageal sphincter. SD, standard deviation (1).

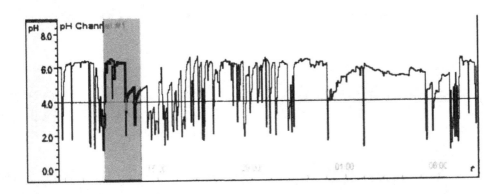

Analysis Results - ch1

Reflux Table - Acid Reflux Analysis

	Meal	Other	Total	Supine	Upright	PrePra	PostPr
Duration of Period (HH: MM)	00:34	02:00	22:21	07:55	14:26	17:47	04:00
Number of Refluxes	13	5	98	11	87	67	18
Number of Long Refluxes(>5 (min))	0	0	7	0	7	7	0
Duration of longest reflux (min)	0	1	23	1	23	23	3
Time pH <4 ((min))	1	2	98	5	92	89	8
Fraction Time pH <4 ((%))	3.7	2.3	7.3	1.2	10.7	8.4	3.4

Figure 5.6 Abnormal acid exposure to the esophagus mostly in the upright position. There were a few episodes of acid exposure during the supine period but these were within the 95th percentile of normal values. The computerized results of the exposure in this test are given in the table and confirm the increased acid exposure in the upright position only.

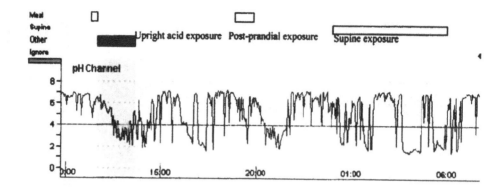

Analysis Results - pH Channel

Acid Period Table

	Total	Uprigt	Supine	Meal	Postpr	Other
Duration of Period	22:05	16:05	06:00	01:20	04:00	02:00
Number of refluxes	331	273	59	8	167	77
Number of long refluxes	6	1	5	0	0	0
Duration of longest reflux (min)	54	23	54	1	4	1
Time pH < 4 (min)	228	105	124	2	46	17
Percent time pH < 4 (%)	17.2	10.8	34.4	3.0	19.2	14.2
Minimum	0.5	0.5	1.3	2.3	1.7	2.1
Maximum	8.6	8.6	7.3	7.2	7.3	7.2
Mean	5.8	6.0	5.1	6.4	5.3	5.4
Median	6.6	6.7	6.4	6.6	5.4	5.7

DeMeester Score (Total): 92.5 DeMeester normals: < 14.72 (95th percentile)

Figure 5.7 A pH recording of a patient who complained of severe heartburn and regurgitation. Abnormal acid exposure was noted in both the erect and supine positions. The DeMeester score was 92.5. The analysis conforms the increased acid exposure (the fraction of time at the pH less than 4 was increased in the upright, supine, and postprandial periods.

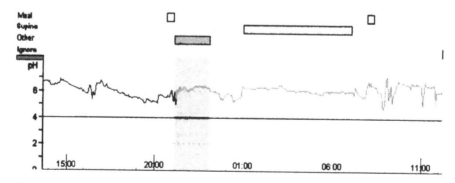

Figure 5.8 A pH recording from a patient who had severe reflux esophagitis. Symptoms were completely relieved following a Nissen fundoplication operation. A postoperative pH study confirmed complete control of all acid exposure to the esophagus.

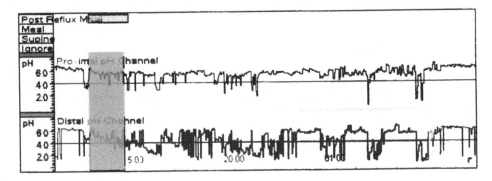

Reflux Table - Proximal

	Total	Upright	Supine	Meal	PostPr	Post Reflux Meal
Duration of Period (HH: MM)	20:56	14:11	06:45	00:47	05:48	02:00
Number of Refluxes	55	45	10	16	27	3
Number of Long Refluxes(>5 (min))	0	0	0	0	0	0
Duration of longest reflux (min)	2	2	2	1	2	1
Time pH <4 ((min))	26	18	8	4	13	2
Fraction Time pH <4 ((%))	2.1	2.1	2.0	8.8	4.0	2.0

DeMeester Score-Proximal

Total score = 10.0 , DeMeester normals less than 14.72 (95th percentile)

Reflux Table - Distal

	Total	Meal	Supine	Upright	PostPr	Other
Duration of Period (HH: MM)	21:11	00:30	06:59	14:11	03:59	02:00
Number of Refluxes	287	4	30	258	62	49
Number of Long Refluxes(>5 (min))	10	0	2	9	2	2
Duration of longest reflux (min)	49	1	12	49	7	7
Time pH <4 ((min))	298	2	36	262	35	30
Fraction Time pH <4 ((%))	23.5	7.8	8.6	30.8	14.9	25.0

DeMeester Score-Distal

Total score = 80.6 , DeMeester normals less than 14.72 (95th percentile)

Figure 5.9 A double pH probe recording in a 30-year-old patient who had suffered from asthma for 15 years. Abnormal upright, supine, and postprandial acid exposure was noted in both the upper and lower esophagus. The analysis of the recordings are shown in the tables.

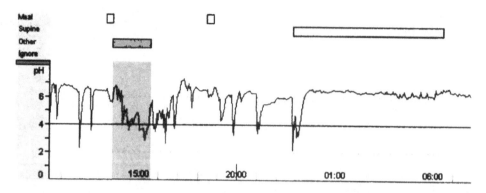

Analysis Results - pH Channel

Acid Period Table

	Total	Uprigt	Supine	Meal	Postpr	Other
Duration of Period	21:40	14:00	07:40	00:40	04:00	02:00
Number of refluxes	94	86	9	1	40	31
Number of long refluxes	5	4	1	0	2	2
Duration of longest reflux (min)	17	17	9	0	17	17
Time pH < 4 (min)	104	87	17	0	47	41
Percent time pH < 4 (%)	8.0	10.4	3.8	0.2	19.4	34.3
Minimum	1.2	1.2	1.3	2.9	2.2	2.2
Maximum	7.5	7.5	6.8	7.1	7.5	7.5
Mean	5.8	5.7	6.1	6.0	5.2	4.7
Median	6.2	6.1	8.3	6.1	5.5	4.5

DeMeester Score (Total): 29.3 DeMeester normals: < 14.72 (95th percentile)

Figure 5.10   A pH recording showing postprandial acid exposure in the esophagus. There is also some upright reflux, but the major contribution to the positive DeMeester score is from the postprandial period.

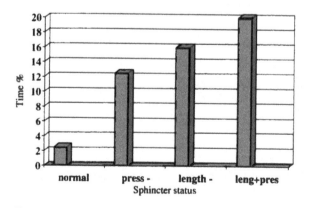

Figure 5.11   Percentage postprandial time for normal subjects, patients with a structurally intact sphincter, and patients with a defective sphincter as determined by inadequate sphincter pressure, length, or a combination of inadequate length and pressure ($P < 0.001$ ANOVA; least significant differences: α vs. all other groups; β vs. normal subjects, structurally intact, and length- and pressure-defective groups; γ vs. normal subjects, structurally intact, and length-only and pressure-only groups; δ vs. all other groups).

REFERENCE

1. Mason RJ, Oberg S, Bremner CG, Peters JH, Gadenstatter M, Ritter M, DeMeester TR. Post-prandial gastroesophageal reflux in normal volunteers and symptomatic patients. J Gastrointest Surg 1998; 2:342–349.

6. CATHETER-FREE AMBULATORY pH MONITORING: HISTORICAL MILESTONES

1957	Jacobson and Mackay developed the pH radiotelemetry capsule.
1964	Connell and Waters studied gastric pH with a radiotelemetry capsule.
1971	Kunz, Norby, and Rogers recorded whole gut pH using a radio capsule.
1972	Kurt and Kang suspended a radiotelemetry capsule in the esophagus to detect gastroesophageal reflux.

REFERENCES

Connell AM, Waters TE. Assessment of gastric function by pH telemetering capsule. Lancet 1964; ii:227–230.

Jacobson B, Mackay RS. A pH—endoradiosonde. Lancet 1957; i:1224.

Kunz HJ, Norby TE, Rogers CH. Dig Dis 1971; 16:739–743.

Kurt EJ, Kang S. Radiotelemetry pH determination for gastroesophageal reflux. Analysis of 521 cases. Am J Gastroenterol 1972; 58(4):390–395.

7. "BRAVO™" PROBE (MEDTRONIC, INC.)

7.1. Equipment

1. The remote probe that lies in the oesophagus is 25 mm × 6 mm × 5.5 mm and contains an antimony pH electrode, a radiotransmitter, and a battery.

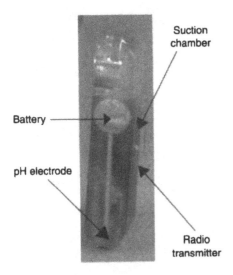

Figure 5.12 Esophageal probe.

2. Esophageal pH is measured every 6 s and two pH data points are transmitted every 12 s to the receiver unit.

A delivery system is required to place the probe in the esophagus and attach it to the mucosa. This consists of a long hollow catheter. The probe is attached to the distal end, and a locking/release plunger and a vacuum port are located at the proximal end in the unit's handle.

Calibration: Details of calibration are provided by the manufacturers.

7.2. Probe Insertion

1. The delivery device is inserted through an anesthetized nostril and the probe positioned appropriately in the esophagus 5 cm above the manometrically deter-mined proximal border of the lower esophageal sphincter. The probe can be positioned via the mouth, which is an easier procedure for the patient, but the accuracy of the method has not been defined. Those who are using the oral technique should position the probe 6 cm above the endoscopically observed position where the mucosal folds of the gastric epithelium end.
2. A vacuum pump is attached to the port on the handle of the delivery device and turned on. This draws a bleb of esophageal mucosa into the probe chamber.
3. Once a steady vacuum has been achieved, the plunger on the handle of the deliv-ery device is depressed to fire a locking pin through the bleb of mucosa, thus securing it to the oesophagus.
4. The vacuum is then released, and the plunger rotated to detach the probe from the delivery device. The latter is then removed from the patient.

The radio receiver unit is 100 mm × 70 mm × 30 mm and weighs 165 g. A clip on the unit's back enables it to be worn on the patient's waist in a similar fashion to a standard telecommunications pager. The upper edge of the unit continuously displays the current time and pH value. Buttons on the outer casing allow the patient to indicate when symp-toms are experienced during the study. Should the patient ever become out of range of their receiver, a high pitched tone sounds. At the conclusion of the study, the information is transferred via an infrared datalink to a personal computer for analysis.

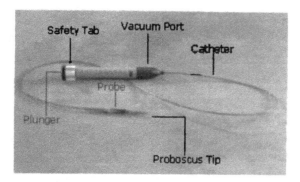

Figure 5.13 Delivery system.

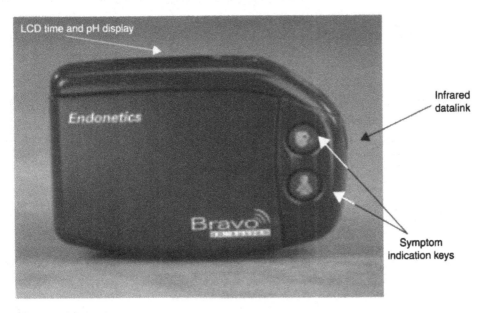

Figure 5.14 Receiver.

7.3. Patient Instructions

The Bravo ambulatory pH study is performed in exactly the same manner as for the catheter-based studies. Therefore, patients need to be informed about stopping medications that affect gastric acid production or esophagogastric motility, adopting dietary restrictions and indicating when they should have meals and lie down to sleep.

7.4. Scoring System

The Bravo probe is physically attached to the esophagus rather than simply being tethered to the nose, as is the case with the catheter-based systems. Because of this, the probe maintains a constant distance from the esophagogastric junction and does not "dip down"

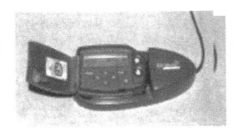
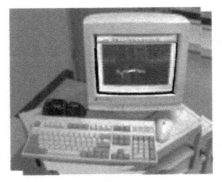

Figure 5.15 Uploading the pH data.

toward the stomach with each swallow-induced shortening of the esophagus. Therefore, it was important to establish a new set of normal values.

The Bravo normal values were derived from 50 asymptomatic volunteers and are listed below.

Table 5.2 "Bravo" Esophageal Acid Exposure in the 1st and 2nd 24 h in 50 Asymptomatic Volunteers

	1st 24 h		2nd 24 h	
	Mean (±SD)	95th percentile	Mean (±SD)	95th percentile
% Total time at pH less than 4	1.79 (2.16)	5.89	1.78 (1.78)	5.64
% Upright time at pH less than 4	2.45 (3.14)	7.81	2.54 (2.57)	7.46
% Supine time at pH less than 4	0.37 (1.18)	1.58	0.34 (1.28)	1.29
Number of Reflux episodes	21.22 (18.59)	55.30	22.31 (19.87)	56.15
Number of Reflux episodes >5 min	0.62 (1.21)	3.55	0.75 (1.15)	3.00
Duration longest reflux episode	3.79 (4.31)	11.23	5.95 (4.52)	17.03
DeMeester score	6.02 (4.82)	15.93	5.95 (4.52)	15.48
% Post-prandial time at pH less than 4	1.72 (3.79)	10.86	1.28 (2.66)	7.63
% Post-challenging (refluxogenic) meal time at pH less than 4	3.85 (6.77)	20.78	3.04 (4.44)	13.92

6
Bilitec Monitoring

1. SPECTROPHOTOMETRY APPARATUS

In the absence of carotene and serum lipids, the bilirubin concentration in a solution can be directly measured by spectrophotometry on the basis of specific absorption at a wavelength of 453 nm. According to Beer's law, absorbance (A) is the logarithm of the ratio between the intensity of light transmitted (I°) through a solution containing an absorbing substance and the intensity of light transmitted (I) in the absence of the absorbing substance: $A = \log(I^{\circ}/I)$.

The apparatus used to measure the presence of bilirubin consists of a portable optoelectronic datalogger, weighing 1200 g, which can be strapped to the patient's side, and a fiberoptic probe which can be passed transnasally and positioned anywhere in the lumen of the foregut (Bilitec: Medtronic, Inc.). The spectrophotometric probes are 3 mm in diameter and 140 cm in length and contain 36 plastic optical fibers, each 250 μm in diameter, bonded together and covered with biocompatible polyurethane. Two plugs connect 50% of the optic fibers to the light emitting diodes and 50% to the receiving photodiode. The tip of the probe contains a 2 mm space for sampling. Fluids and blenderized solids can easily flow through the space and their bilirubin concentration are measured. The probes are flexible, durable, easy to sterilize, and reusable.

The optoelectronic unit acts simultaneously as a light signal generator, a data processor, and a data storage device (1,2). The unit has two channels allowing dual measurement with two probes if desired. The light source for each channel is provided by two light emitting diodes, which emit a 470 nm signal light (blue spectrum) and a 565 nm reference light (green spectrum). Reference and signal light emitting diodes are stimulated alternately for a duration of 0.5 s. To avoid fluctuations in the source, the final 20 ms of each pulse is used for signal processing. Optical signals reflected back from the probe are converted to electrical impulses by a photodiode. This electrical signal is then amplified and processed within the datalogger (80 C196KC, Intel, California). Absorbance readings are averaged every two cycles. The system is capable of recording 225 individual absorbance values per hour and allows up to 30 h of continuous monitoring.

REFERENCES

1. Bechi P, Pucciani F, Baldini F et al. Long-term ambulatory enterogastric reflux monitoring. Validation of a new fiberoptic technique. Dig Dis Sci 1993; 38:1297–1306.
2. Kauer WKH, Burdiles P, Ireland AP, Clark GWB, Peters JH, Bremner CG, DeMeester TR. Does duodenal juice reflux into the esophagus of patients with complicated GERD? Evaluation of a fiberoptic sensor for bilirubin. Am J Surg 1995; 169:98–104.

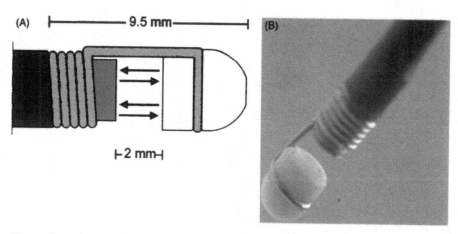

Figure 6.1 The tip of the fiberoptic probe has a 2 mm space for sampling. Fluid can easily move into and out of the space and the presence of bilirubin can be detected by its absorbance. The pH probe to the right compares the size. A pH probe and a Bilitec probe can be used together to measure acid and bilirubin exposure.

2. PATIENT INSTRUCTIONS

2.1. Foods that Can Be Eaten for the Bilitec 2000 Study

1. Bananas
2. Apples
3. Saltine crackers
4. Cottage cheese
5. Chicken breast, baked, broiled, and boiled—no skin
6. Rice
7. Cream of chicken or cream of mushroom soup

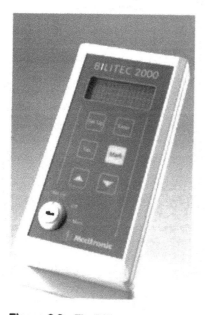

Figure 6.2 The Bilitec recorder.

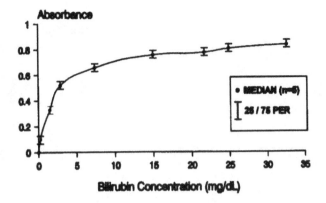

Figure 6.3   Correlation between absorbance and bilirubin concentration.

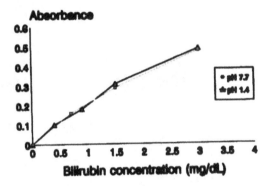

Figure 6.4   Effect of pH on bilirubin absorbance.

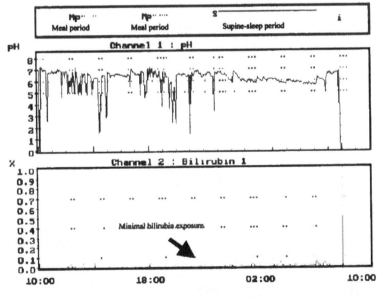

Figure 6.5   Upper recording demonstrates a pH recording. Lower recording demonstrates bilirubin exposure. Both recordings are within normal ranges. There is no bilirubin above 0.1 in this recording. Mp, meal period; S, supine period.

8. Bread
9. Boiled noodles/pasta (may use parmesan cheese to flavor, white cheeses, i.e., mozzarella, monterey jack, swiss, or alfredo sauce)
10. Potatoes, baked, boiled, or mashed—no skin
11. Cream of wheat or rice
12. Vanilla ice cream
13. Lowfat milk
14. Water

Only low fat milk or water to drink. No soda pop, coffee, tea, alcohol, or candy. No butter or margarine.

This test depends on the patient not eating anything green or yellow or anything that may have green or yellow substances in it. The machine uses a special technique that measures the color of the juice that is coming back in the esophagus. Patients must document all the things that are eaten.

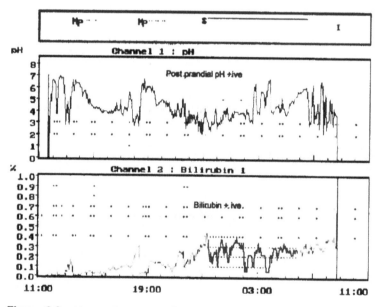

Figure 6.6 Abnormal exposure of both acid and bilirubin in the upright and supine periods.

Drown

HIGH EPISODE (CHANNEL 2)		Total	Upright	Supine	Meal
Duration	(HH:MM)	22:04	13:39	08:25	00:37
Number of episodes	(#)	294	91	204	0
Number of episodes					
longer than 5.0 minutes	(#)	7	3	4	0
Longest episode	(min)	48	20	48	0
Total time Bilirubin 1 above 0.20	(min)	207	72	135	0
Fraction time Bilirubin 1 above 0.20	(%)	15.6	8.8	26.7	0.0

Figure 6.7 Tabulated results of the recording confirms the abnormal exposure in the upright and supine periods.

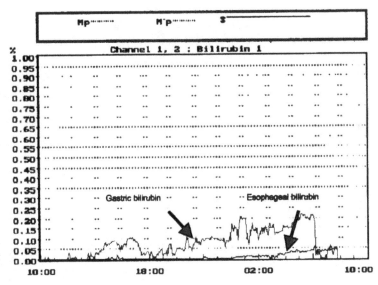

Figure 6.8 Combined gastric and esophageal bilirubin study. Gastric exposure reaches the 0.2 level and esophageal exposure is minimal. Both results are within normal limits.

3. NORMAL VALUES FOR ESOPHAGEAL EXPOSURE TO BILIRUBIN (35 HEALTHY VOLUNTEERS)

The median percentage time with absorbance greater than 0.2 is 0%, the 75th percentile is 0.1%, the 95th percentile is 1.7% and the 99th percentile is 6.7% (1).

In a study by Cuomo et al. (2) the total bilirubin absorbance above 0.14 (absorbance × min) was 7.8 ± 2.2 in patients without esophagitis, 11.7 ± 4.4 in patients with Grade I–II esophagitis, and 17 ± 4.2 in patients with Grade III–IV esophagitis.

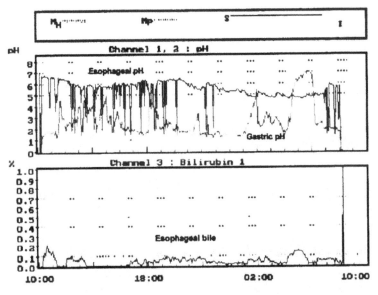

Figure 6.9 Combined esophageal and gastric pH studies with esophageal bilitec recording (normal ranges).

In vitro correlation studies. Vaezi et al. (3) found a strong correlation between Bilitec absorption in 63 samples of bilirubin ditaurate and human bile ($R = 0.82$). The correlation was less strong in an acid medium with a pH of 3.5. Cuomo et al. (2) found only minor effect of acid on absorption when studying esophageal acid and bilirubin exposure in patients.

4. PATTERNS OF COMBINED ESOPHAGEAL AND GASTRIC BILITEC RECORDING

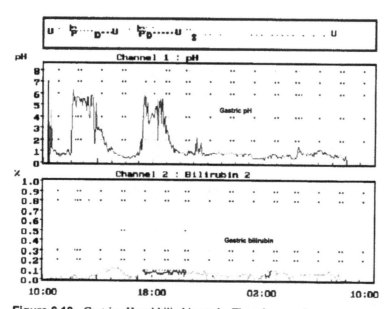

Figure 6.10 Gastric pH and bilirubin study. There is normal exposure.

Table 6.1 Normal Values for Gastric Bilirubin Exposure

Absorbance	Mean ± SD	Median	95th percentile
>0.14	24.2 ± 20.7	20.3	62.3
>0.2	11.6 ± 11.5	8.1	33.4
>0.25	6.8 ± 7.9	4.3	24.8
>0.3	4.0 ± 5.6	1	14.3
>0.4	1.7 ± 2.7	0.2	7.4

Source: After Fein et al. Dig Dis Sci 2002; 2769–2774.

Table 6.2 Gastric Bilirubin Studies. Absorbance Threshold 0.25% Time

Billroth 1 gastrectomy	$n = 5$	29 ± 4.3
Billroth 11 gastrectomy	$n = 15$	60.1 ± 24
Roux-en-Y	$n = 9$	21.7 ± 38.2
Cholecystectomy	$n = 25$	27.9 ± 24.6
Failed antireflux surgery	$n = 14$	22.0 ± 16

Source: After Fein et al. Dig Dis Sci 2002; 2769–2774.

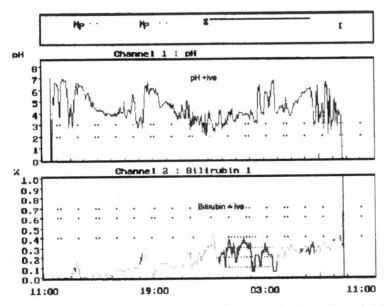

Figure 6.11 Esophageal pH and gastric bilirubin. During the supine period there was esophageal acid exposure and a surge of bile into the stomach.

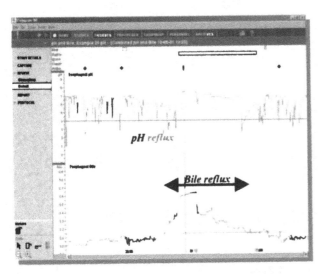

Figure 6.12 Esophageal pH and Bilitec study. Maximal bile reflux has occurred during the supine period. Note that there is also acid exposure in the esophagus during the upright and supine periods.

REFERENCES

1. Fein M, Ireland AP, Ritter MP, Peters JH, Hagen JA, Bremner CG, DeMeester TR. Duodenogastric reflux potentiates the injurious effects of gastroesophageal reflux. J Gastrointest Surg 1997; 1:27–33.

2. Cuomo R, Koek G, Sifrim D, Janssens J, Tack J. Analysis of ambulatory duodeno gastroeso-phageal reflux monitoring. Dig Dis Sci 2002; 45(12):2463–2469.
3. Vaezi MF, Lacemera RG, Richter JE. Validation studies of Bilitec 2000: an ambulatory duodenogastric monitoring system. Am J Physiol 1994; 267(6 Pt 1):G1050–G1057.

7
Esophageal Impedance

1. ESOPHAGEAL IMPEDANCE (IMPEDANCOMETRY)

Definition. Esophageal impedance is a measure of the resistance to electrical conductivity of the esophagus and its contents, and is used to measure bolus transport. Impedance is inversely proportional to electrical conductivity.

Measurement. A small AC voltage is applied to two electrodes on a catheter assembly. This generates a small current that is proportional to the conductivity of the esophagus and its contents. When the esophagus is empty and relaxed the impedance is high, but when a bolus expands the esophagus, the impedance is low. The electrical current is so small that it does not affect the esophageal neuromuscular mechanism.

Esophageal impedance combined with motility and reflux monitoring (Multichannel intraluminal impedance, MII, Sandhill Scientific Inc.). A single catheter incorporates electrodes for impedance measurement, transducers for pressure measurement, and a pH probe.

1.1. Clinical Uses

1. Measurement of all types of gastroesophageal reflux (i.e., acid and non-acid refluxates, liquid or gas and mixed refluxates) (1,2);
2. Assessment of high gastroesophageal reflux;
3. Measurement of swallow function by bolus transport;
4. Assessment of patients for GERD therapy, that is, suitability for endoscopic or operative antireflux procedure;
5. Identification of patients "at risk" for fundoplication, because of poor bolus transport;
6. Assessment of patients with dysphagia, inadequate esophageal motility (IEM), and precordial chest pain;
7. Assessment of recurrent symptoms after antireflux symptoms.

1.2. Catheter Design

Three catheters are available:

1. Adult model with esophageal pH probe;
2. Adult model with esophageal and gastric pH probes;
3. Pediatric model.

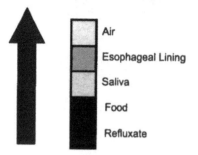

Low Conductivity = High impedance

Air

Esophageal Lining

Saliva

Food

Refluxate

High Conductivity = Low impedance

Figure 7.1 Impedance scale: refluxate has a high conductivity and a low impedance. Air has a low conductivity and a high impedance.

1.3. EFT Protocol

Ten saline swallows.

Ten viscous swallows (viscous swallow challenge approximates food intake). Viscous is supplied in various flavors.

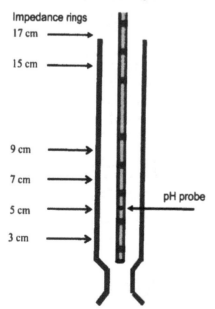

Standard Adult ComforTEC® GER and pH monitoring catheter

Impedance rings

17 cm

15 cm

9 cm

7 cm

5 cm

3 cm

pH probe

Figure 7.2 The esophageal function test (EFT) catheter. Impedance probes are at levels 17, 15, 9, 7, 5, and 3 cm from the catheter tip. A pH probe is at the 5 cm level.

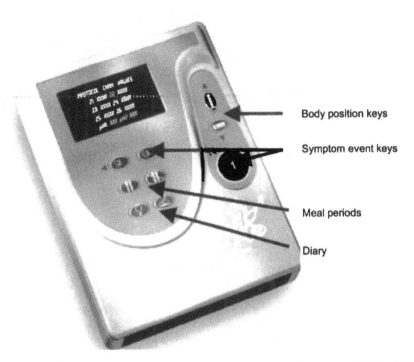

Figure 7.3 "Sleuth" monitor is attached to the catheter and worn around a belt during the recording period.

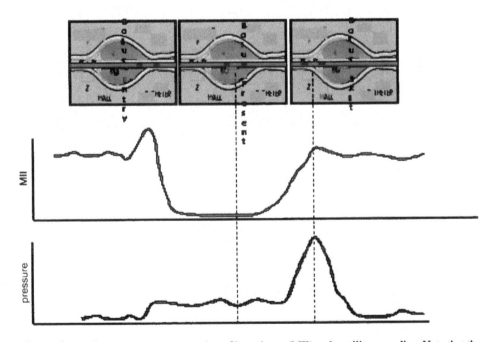

Figure 7.4 Diagrammatic representation of impedance (MII) and motility recording. Note that the empty esophagus has a high impedance, and when it is filled with fluid, the impedance decreases. The impedance waveform is opposite to the contraction waveform. The bolus exit point occurs in front of the contraction wave.

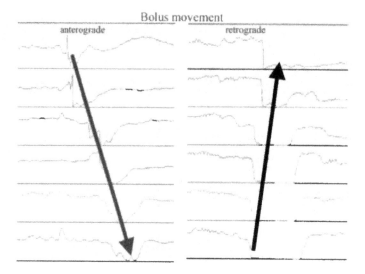

Figure 7.5   Antegrade and retrograde bolus transport. (Left) As the bolus moves down the esophagus there is a sequential change in the impedance recording ("peristaltic" appearance but the deflections are reversed in comparison to the deflections seen on manometry). (Right) The deflections are reversed from below upwards because the bolus is moving in a retrograde direction.

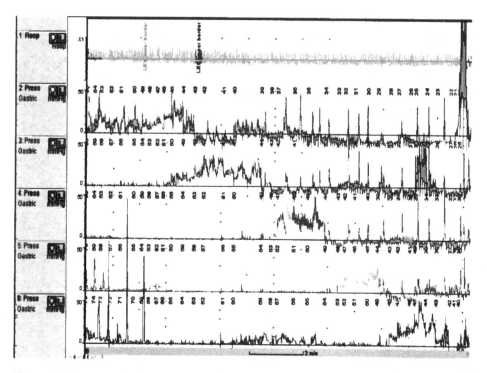

Figure 7.6   EFT study. A stationary pull-through study of the lower esophageal sphincter (LES). Five channels have recorded the LES. The record has been compressed and can be expanded for a detailed view of the LES, which can be assessed using the same methods as described in the section on the LES.

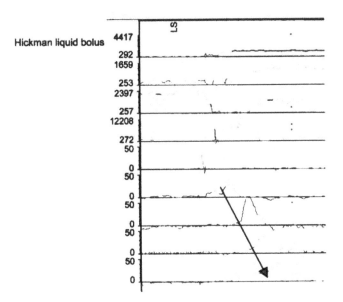

Hickman liquid bolus

Figure 7.7 A liquid bolus study. The upper four channels have recorded the impedance characteristics of the swallow. The lower four channels are the corresponding pressure responses to the swallow.

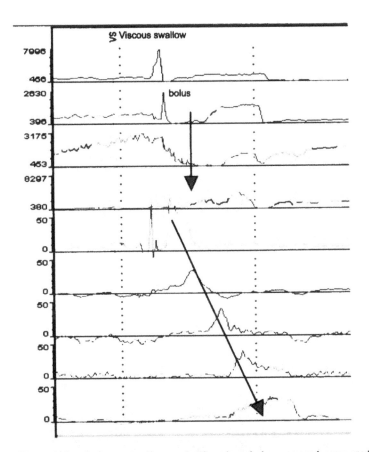

Figure 7.8 A viscous swallow study. Note that a bolus pressure is generated by the viscous swallow.

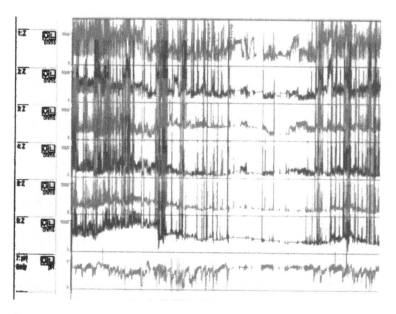

Figure 7.9   A compressed recording of a 24 h impedance and pH study. This compressed recording can be expanded to read any section of the record from 2 min intervals and upwards.

1.4.   Bolus Clearance Patterns

Manometry gives a poor prediction of bolus transport.

1.   Bolus clearance: Time elapsed from bolus entry to physical clearance of
     swallowed material.
2.   Acid clearance. Time pH is less than 4. Manometry may show ineffective
     peristalsis, but impedance studies may show complete bolus transport and
     vice versa.

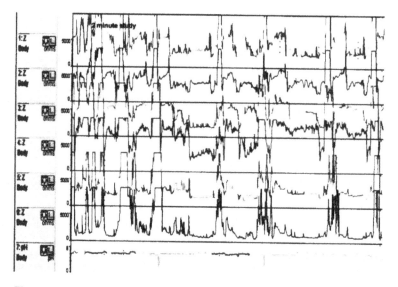

Figure 7.10   A 2 min recording from the above record.

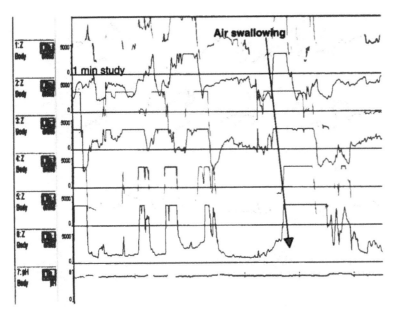

Figure 7.11 An expanded recording of the same study to show details of normal swallowing and air swallowing in six channels and a pH recording in the last channel. Note that the liquid bolus causes a drop in the impedance, whereas the air bolus raises the impedance.

1.5. Data Acquisition

The "Sleuth acquisition Data Program" (Sandhill Scientific Inc.) will record data related to patient position, mealtimes, and symptoms.

The software includes an "AutoSCAN" component which (1) locates waveform areas with retrograde bolus movements; (2) determines bolus entry and clearance points when reflux occurs; and (3) analyzes the pH channel to determine when the pH drops below 4.

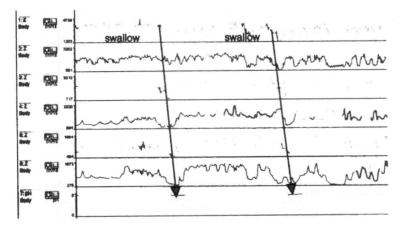

Figure 7.12 Impedance recording of two normal swallows and a normal pH recording.

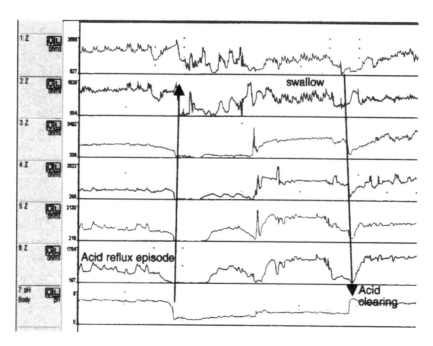

Figure 7.13 Impedance detection of an acid reflux episode (note the pH drop below 4 in the last channel). Following two subsequent swallows there is acid clearing to a pH above 4. Swallow, antegrade transmission; Burp, simultaneous retrograde transmission.

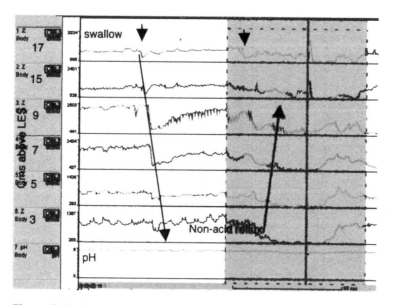

Figure 7.14 Impedance detection of nonacid reflux. The pH probe detected a refluxate of nonacid material. This reflux episode extended to the proximal probe.

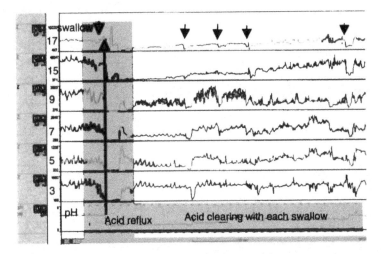

Figure 7.15 Impedance detection of acid reflux. Impedance is recorded in the five channels below the swallow channel. The pH probe of last channel has detected a drop in pH less than 4, indicating acid reflux which extends to 17 cm above the LES. Note the acid clearing that takes place with each swallow.

2. BOLUS TRANSPORT

2.1. Normal Values

Normal values of BTT are as follows:

> Saline swallows <12 s, >80% complete.
> Viscous swallows <13 s, >70% complete.

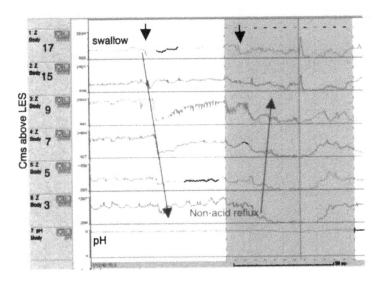

Figure 7.16 Impedance detection of nonacid reflux. The pH probe detected a refluxate of nonacid material. This reflux extended to the proximal probe.

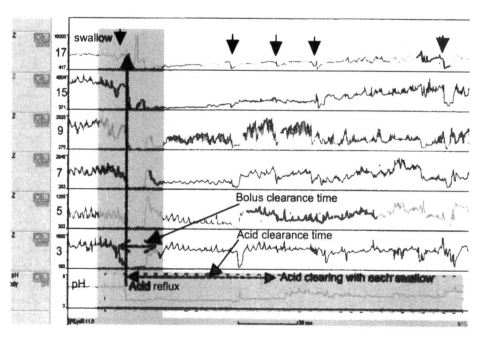

Figure 7.17 Acid reflux. Bolus clearance time and acid clearance times were measured.

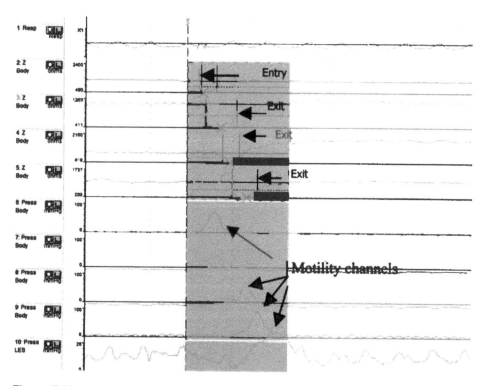

Figure 7.18 Complete bolus transport. The bolus enters impedance channel 1 and exits impedance channels 2, 3, and 4. Note the simultaneous manometric recording in channels 6–10 showing normal motility.

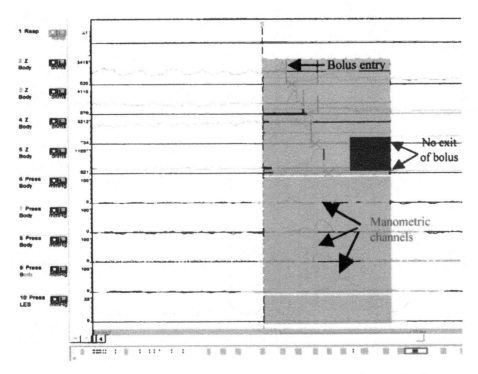

Figure 7.19 Incomplete bolus transport. The bolus did not exit from channels 3 and 4.

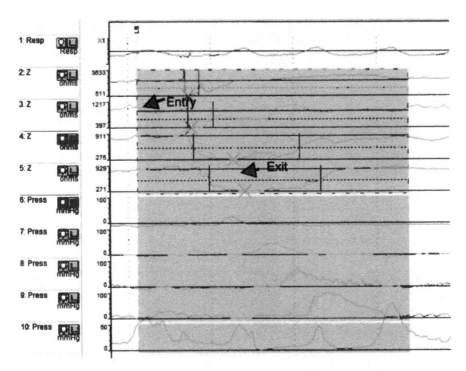

Figure 7.20 Measurement of total bolus transport time. The time elapsed from bolus entry at impedance channel 1 to exit at impedance channel 4 is the bolus transit time (BTT). In this example it is 8.2 s.

3. ANIMATED DISPLAY OF SWALLOW EVENTS

This programme includes an interesting animation display of swallow events which will demonstrate normal bolus transport, escape of the bolus, and reflux events.

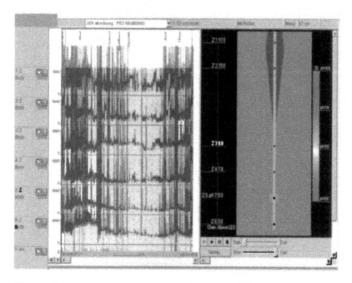

Figure 7.21 An area of interest was selected (shaded area). When the animation starts, the cursor (seen in the left one-third of the shaded area) moves from left to right across the selected area. Simultaneously the animation profile on the right side of this picture depicts the passage of the bolus down the esophagus (see the contraction wave which indents the edge of the lumen). The impedance profile is depicted in the central dark area of the picture. Channels marked 1–4 are impedance channels. Channels marked 5–9 are pressure channels.

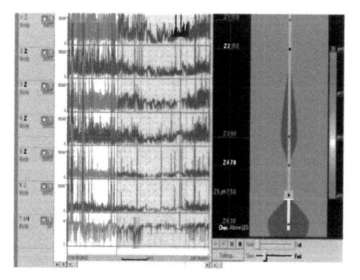

Figure 7.22 As the cursor moves from left to right the bolus indentation and the impedance profiles change. The animation can be used on any section of the swallow recording.

REFERENCES

Balaji N, Peters JH, Gurski R, Gattolin A, Theodorou D, Antonniazi L, DeMeester SL, Hagen JA, Crookes PF, Sillin L, Bremner CG, DeMeester TR. Gas-associated gastroesophageal reflux and its contribution to the spectrum of gastroesophageal reflux. Gastroenterology 2002; 122(4):A338.

Vela MF, Camacho-Lobato C, Srinivasan R, Tutian R, Katz PO, Castell DO. Simultaneous intra-esophageal impedance and pH measurement of acid and non-acid gastro-esophageal reflux. Effect of omeprazole. Gastroenterology 2001; 120:1599–1606.

Index